MEDICAL SPANISH

Fourth Edition

GAIL L. BONGIOVANNI, M.D.

MCGRAW-HILL
Medical Publishing Division

New York   Chicago   San Francisco   Lisbon   London   Madrid
Mexico City   Milan   New Delhi   San Juan   Seoul   Singapore
Sydney   Toronto

Medical Spanish, Fourth Edition

1 2 3 4 5 6 7 8 9 0 DOC/DOC 0 9 8 7 6 5

ISBN: 0-07-144200-6

This book was set in Souvenir by Matrix Publishing Services.
The editors were Janet Foltin, Robert Pancotti, and Patrick Carr.
The production supervisor was Richard Ruzycka.
The cover designer was Aimee Nordin.
The indexer was Janet Perlman.
RR Donnelley was printer and binder.

This book is printed on acid-free paper.

Library of Congress Cataloging-in-Publication Data

Bongiovanni, Gail.
    Medical Spanish / Gail L. Bongiovanni.—4th ed.
      p. cm.
    Includes index.
    ISBN 0-07-144200-6
      1. Spanish language—Conversation and phrase books (for medical personnel) I. Title.
    PC4120.M3B6 2005
    468.3′421′02461—dc22

                                    2004065618

MEDICAL
SPANISH

NOTICE

Medicine is an ever-changing science. As new research and clinical experience broaden our knowledge, changes in treatment and drug therapy are required. The authors and the publisher of this work have checked with sources believed to be reliable in their efforts to provide information that is complete and generally in accord with the standards accepted at the time of publication. However, in view of the possibility of human error or changes in medical sciences, neither the editors nor the publisher nor any other party who has been involved in the preparation or publication of this work warrants that the information contained herein is in every respect accurate or complete, and they disclaim all responsibility for any errors or omissions or for the results obtained from use of the information contained in this work. Readers are encouraged to confirm the information contained herein with other sources. For example and in particular, readers are advised to check the product information sheet included in the package of each drug they plan to administer to be certain that the information contained in this work is accurate and that changes have not been made in the recommended dose or in the contraindications for administration. This recommendation is of particular importance in connection with new or infrequently used drugs.

To My Parents . . . because of the
love and respect we share.

Contents

Preface

I am pleased to present the fourth edition of *Medical Spanish*. With the growing number of Spanish-speaking people now living in the United States, it is timely to have a book that will facilitate comprehensive medical care for the Spanish-speaking patient.

Since the first publication in 1978, *Medical Spanish* has assisted English-speaking medical personnel as they tried to communicate and administer health care to their Spanish-speaking patients.

This fourth edition of *Medical Spanish* continues the comprehensive yet simple linguistic approach that allows medical personnel to take a thorough medical history and perform a complete medical examination on their Spanish-speaking patients.

In this edition I have added new sections on patient privacy issues and breast feeding. There is a revised and expanded chapter on birth control and another on HIV. The new Chapter 11 covers issues of physical and sexual abuse and rape.

My special gratitude to Dr. Molly Katz for her expert guidance on Chapter 9, Contraception and Patient Instruction; Chapter 10, Pregnancy and Delivery; and Chapter 11, Physical and Sexual Abuse and Rape.

My appreciation to Ms. Teresita Lewis for her secretarial and linguistic assistance during the preparation of this edition.

Once again it is my privilege to thank the people of Spain and of all of Latin America for sharing their language and love of life with me since 1967.

MEDICAL
SPANISH

Chapter 1
HOW TO USE
THIS BOOK

Medical Spanish, formerly entitled *Entre doctor y paciente*,[1] was written to aid English-speaking medical personnel working with Spanish-speaking patients. This book is intended to provide a practical method for improving communication.

This book was originally prepared in Guatemala City, Guatemala. Practical trials were carried out for two months at Roosevelt Hospital, Guatemala City, where effectiveness of the text was tested in patient interviews.

1.1   ENGLISH INTO SPANISH

The vocabulary presented is representative of Spanish as it is spoken in Spain and Latin America. The English phrases have not always been given a literal translation. Instead, the Spanish words and phrases have been chosen to communicate the sense

---

[1]*Between Doctor and Patient.*

1

of the English questions in a way that will be understood by the patient.

Example:

I am going to examine   Voy a examinarle su . . .
your . . .

1 abdomen.   1 *estómago* (stomach).

Here the English word "abdomen" is translated as "estómago" (stomach). Wherever such free translating is done, the words involved are marked by an asterisk, and the literal translation of the Spanish word is given in parentheses. In this way, the interviewer will not read one word in English and think the same word has been translated literally into Spanish.

In order to keep the English and the Spanish phrases structurally similar, it was necessary, in some instances, to use a slightly awkward English wording. The Spanish phrase, however, is worded correctly and naturally.

Example:

Is the diarrhea . . .   La diarrea es . . .

1 of what color?   1 de qué color?
2 with blood?   2 con sangre?
3 with fat?   3 con grasa?

Thus, if interviewers follow the Spanish translation presented in the text, they will be speaking grammatically and idiomatically.

1.2 ORGANIZATION OF THE BOOK

The text is divided into fifteen chapters. Several chapters have been subdivided into sections to facilitate the collection of information. For the chapters on review of systems and physical examination, each section is devoted to one organ system. Certain sections have been further subdivided.

Example:

Chapter 5 Chief Complaint or Review of Systems
Section 5.4 Gastrointestinal System
Section 5.4.1 Nutritional History

Chapter 2 introduces some essentials of Spanish grammar. The Appendix presents basic and supplemental vocabulary.

The remainder of the text is to be used during an interview with a patient who comes to the clinic or hospital. The interview begins with questions about the patient's social and economic history. Patient privacy issues are also presented in this chapter (Chapter 3). Questions on past medical history, review of systems, physical examination, general treatment and follow-up, and medical therapy are covered in Chapters 4 to 8. Four special chapters cover topics of contraception, labor and delivery, physical abuse and rape, and poisonings. Psychiatric evaluation and geriatric assessment are each separate chapters.

1.3 THE INTERVIEW FORMAT

For the interviewer with little knowledge of Spanish, a response to an open-ended question may be difficult to understand. To avoid confusion, the questions to the patient hava been phrased so that they can be answered either "Yes" ("Si") or "No"("No"). Several variations on the yes/no question are also used. To round out the interview, a multipurpose request format, which is to be accompanied by appropriate gestures, is provided.

1.3.1 Basic Yes/No Question

Almost all questions in this book are phrased so that the patient may answer "Si" or "No" as the interviewer reads them. Some questions begin with a repeating phrase to which a list of different words or phrases may be appended.

Example:

Do you often . . .   Tiene *frecuentemente* . . .

1 feel nauseated?   1 *náusea?*
2 vomit?   2 *vómitos?*
3 burp?   3 *eructos?*

The interviewer is not supposed to suggest symptoms to the patient. He simply asks, "Do you often feel *nauseated?* and *waits* for the patient to respond "Si" or "No". Other questions give more detailed information, but the basic format is the same.

Example:

Do you have pain on urination . . .	Tiene *dolor* al orinar . . .

1 at the beginning?	1 al *empezar*?
2 the whole time?	2 *todo* el tiempo?
3 at the end?	3 al *terminar*?

This method may alter the usual dialogue between health worker and patient, but it also helps the interviewer obtain information. If the traditional "open-ended" question form is used, it is difficult to restrain the patient from speaking too rapidly, and the interviewer with a limited acquaintance with Spanish will be unable to understand the response.

Three variations of the yes/no question are also employed.

1.3.2 Double-Tense Question

This question format is very practical for someone just learning Spanish. By substituting verb tenses, the interviewer can use the "double-tense questions" to obtain twice as much information. With this method of questioning either the *chief complaint* or *review of systems* (Chapter 5) can be investigated. The interviewer uses the same questions, but changes the tense.

Example:

Do you have OR have you had . . .	Tiene O ha tenido . . .

1 pain in your chest?	1 dolor del pecho?
2 shortness of breath?	2 sensación de ahogo?
3 difficulty in breathing?	3 dificultad al respirar?
4 night sweats?	4 sudor por la noche?

This technique is easy to use and does not require the interviewer to learn a completely new vocabulary. In a very few instances, a question is illogical in one tense. The interviewer should be alert to this possibility and carefully select the tense to be used. The interviewer should not ask "Do you have or have you had. . . ." If the chief complaint is under investigation, the interviewer asks, "Do you have. . . ." If the review of systems is being covered, the interviewer chooses "Have you had. . . ."

1.3.3 One-Common-Phrase Question

Another variation of the basic yes/no question format is the one-common-phrase question. In this variation, the same introductory phrase is used with different words to elicit additional information.

Example:

Have you ever been hit in the . . .	Se ha *golpeado* en . . .
1 head?	1 la cabeza?
2 face?	2 la cara?
3 neck?	3 el cuello?
4 eyes?	4 los ojos?

This question format may change the usual dialogue between health worker and patient but, again, it does simplify and perhaps eliminate the difficulty an English-speaking person may experience in interpreting a Spanish answer.

1.3.4 Fill-In-the-Blank Question

This question format is a version of the one-common-phrase approach. On the basis of responses made previously by the patient, the interviewer can gain additional information simply by substituting the known information into the question.

Example:

In reviewing the cardiovascular system, the interviewer has learned that the patient has experienced "shortness of breath." To obtain additional information about this symptom, the blank in the question is filled in with the known symptom.

Was (Is) the *shortness of breath* accompanied by . . .	Además de la *sensación de ahogo*, tuvo (tiene) . . .
1 fever?	1 *fiebre?*
2 trembling?	2 *temblores?*
3 sweating?	3 *sudores?*

In this example, the combined used of the double-tense question and the fill-in-the blank question provides the interviewer with more extensive information on the patient's problem.

1.3.5 The Multipurpose Request

This request format allows the examiner to communicate several different instructions with the same phrase. This type of presentation is particularly helpful during the physical examination. When using these questions, the interviewer must *actively point to or demonstrate* a particular item.

Example:

Please . . .	Por favor . . .
1 walk on THIS.	1 camine sobre ESTO.

This refers to a treadmill for the exercise tolerance test,

2 take THESE pills.	2 tome ESTAS pildoras.

These refers to a specific color or shape of pills.

Whenever the multipurpose request is used in the book, the variable is shown in capitals as in the examples shown here.

The yes/no question, together with its variations, and the multipurpose request are employed to facilitate the interview, physical examination, and follow-up. This method of interviewing is simple and requires only that the interviewer be a more active participant in the clinic or a hospital visit. For those health workers with a greater knowledge of Spanish, the book provides an ample medical vocabulary, and it should not be difficult for such workers to incorporate the new vocabulary into their usual interview.

Effective communication in a linguistically simple style is the principal goal of this book. The interview format has been designed to minimize the interviewer's difficulty as he or she attempts to communicate in a new language with patients. The primary aim of *Medical Spanish* is to help the English-speaking health worker provide more reassuring and effective health care to Spanish-speaking patients.

Chapter 2
GRAMMAR AND PRONUNCIATION

This book is not intended to provide complete grammatical information. Therefore, there are only a few concepts to keep in mind about grammar and pronunciation.

The syllabic breakdown of the Spanish words is not given. It is recommended that the words be pronounced as they would be in English, keeping the few pronunciation rules in mind. The patient will understand even though the accent may not be perfect.

2.1 PRONUNCIATION

1 Spanish vowels:
   a   is pronounced like "a" in *fAther*.
   e   is pronounced like "ai" in *AIr*.
   i   is pronounced like "ee" in *frEE*.
   o   is pronounced like "o" in *lOw*.
   u   is pronounced like "oe" in *shOE*.
2 When "a," "e," or "o" is followed by "u" or "i," the two vowels form a single sound with prolongation of the "a," "e," or "o" sound.

Example: causa (cause)[1]

When "i" or "u" precedes another vowel, the two vowels form one sound with slight emphasis of the second vowel. *Example:* viuda (widow)

3   "B" and "v" are pronounced exactly alike in Spanish. They sound like the "b" in *aBolition*.

4   "Ch" is an independent letter of the alphabet and is pronounced like the hard "ch" in *CHeese*.

5   At the beginning of a word, "d" is like the hard "d" in *day*. In the middle of a word, "d" is pronounced like the "th" in *wiTH*.
    Example: Todo (all) is pronounced "to-tho."

6   In Spanish the "h" is *always* silent.
    Example: Hijo (son) is pronounced "ee-ho." All other letters are pronounced.

7   "J" is similar to the hard "h" in *horizon* and is slightly guttural.
    Example: Joven (young) is pronounced "ho-ven."

8   A "ll" is pronounced like "ye" in *YEllow*.
    Example: Llamar (call) is pronounced "ya-mar."

9   "Ñ" is a separate letter of the alphabet. It is pronounced like "ny" of *caNYon* and is nasal-sounding.

10 Single "r" at the beginning of a word and "rr" in the middle of a word are always trilled. This sound is made by vibrating the tongue against the roof of the mouth with a strong expulsion of breath.

11 If a word ends in a consonant other than "n" or "s," the stress is on the last syllable.
    Example: ard<u>or</u> (burning)
    Words ending in a vowel, "n," or "s" stress the second to the last syllable.

---

[1]The English translation is always enclosed in parentheses.

Example: ca<u>mi</u>sa (shirt), <u>ca</u>sas (houses)

Any word whose pronunciation differs from these rules will always have a *written accent*.

Example: médico (doctor), not medico.

2.2 GRAMMAR

1 Plurals of nouns are formed simply by adding "s" if the word ends in an unaccented vowel.

Example: dedo (finger)
        dedos (fingers)

or by adding "es" if it ends in a consonant, "y," or an accented vowel.

Example: dolor (pain)
        dolores (pains)
        ley (law)
        leyes (laws)
        rubí (ruby)
        rubíes (rubies)

2 The definite articles are:

Feminine		**Masculine**	
Singular	Plural	Singular	Plural
la	las	el	los

Example: la pierna (the leg)
        las piernas (the legs)
        el brazo (the arm)
        los brazos (the arms)

3 In general, words ending in "o" are masculine and those ending in "a" are feminine. An adjective agrees in number and in gender with the noun it modifies.

Example: niña (girl)   las niñas enfermas (the sick girls)
niño (boy)   el niño enfermo (the sick boy)

One relevant exception to this rule is la mano (the hand) rather than el mano.

4 *Possessive Adjectives*: Unless you are speaking to a child, you should use the formal address.

	Singular	*Plural*
(my)	mi	mis
(your familiar)	tu	tus
(his, her, your formal)	su	sus
(our)	nuestro (a)[2]	nuestros (as)[3]
(your familiar)	vuestro (a)	vuestros (as)
(their)	su	sus

For parts of the body the possessive adjective can be replaced by the definite article. The meaning of the sentence remains clear.

Example: Levante su brazo. (Raise your arm.)

or

Levante el brazo. (still understood as, Raise your arm.)

5 *Subject Pronouns*

	Singular		*Plural*
(I)	yo	(we)	nosotros (as)
(you familiar)	tú	(you familiar)	vosotros (as)
(he)	él[4]	(they)	ellos (as)
(she)	ella		
(you formal)	usted[5]	(you formal)	ustedes

It is not always necessary to write the subject pronoun in a sentence. The conjugated verb is enough.

Example: Yo soy el médico. (I am the doctor.) can correctly be written, Soy el médico.

6 *Contractions*

al = a + el (to the)

del = de + el (of the) It also forms the possessive.

Example: Voy al hospital. (I am going to the hospital.)

la herida del paciente (the patient's wound)

(the wound *of the* patient)

---

[2] The feminine form is made by changing the final "o" to an "a."
[3] The plural is formed by adding "s."
[4] Notice the written accent on él (he) to distinguish it from el (the).
[5] Usted is abbreviated Vd., ustedes is abbreviated Vds.

7   *Common Suffixes and Prefixes*
   a   *Diminutives:* "ito" (a) dolor (pain)
                               dolorcito (slight pain)
   b   *Augmentatives:* "isimo" (a) cansado (tired)
                                cansadísimo (very tired)
   c   *Adverbs:* "mente" is added to the feminine form of the
       adjective to form the adverb.
       generosa (generous)
       generosamente (generously)
   d   *"Dad" and "tad"* are equivalent to the English "ty."
       cantidad (quantity)
       facultad (faculty)
   e   *"Ería"* denotes the location where something is made or
       sold.
       libro (book)
       librería (bookstore)
   f   *"Ero"* (a) indicates the person who makes or sells the ob-
       ject.
       zapato (shoe)
       zapatero (shoemaker)
   g   *"Des"* before a word forms the opposite of the original
       word.
       vestir (to dress)
       desvestir (to undress)
       agradable (agreeable)
       desagradable (disagreeable)

2.3   SPELLING

To spell any word in Spanish, write it exactly as it sounds, re-
membering that the "h" is silent. Normally, only three letters
may be doubled in Spanish:

c   contracción (contraction)
l   ella (she)
r   hierro (iron)

Chapter 3
SOCIAL, ECONOMIC AND PATIENT PRIVACY INFORMATION

3.1   GENERAL SOCIAL BACKGROUND

What is your name?
How old are you?
Where were you born?
When did you come to
this country?
Where do you live?
How long have you lived
there?
What is your address?
Have you lived in _____?[2]
Do you live alone?

DATOS SOCIALES GENERALES

Como se llama usted?[1]
Cuántos años tiene?
Dónde nació?
Cuando vino usted a
este país?
Dónde vive?
Hace cuánto tiempo que
vive allí?
Cuál es su dirección?
Vivió usted en _____?[2]
Vive solo (a)?

[1]For the sake of simplicity, the inverted question mark, which should precede every question, has been omitted.
[2]See index of countries, page 186.

Do you live with your . . .	Vive con . . .
1 parents?	1 sus padres?
2 husband (wife)?	2 su esposo (a)?
3 son (daughter)?	3 su hijo (a)?
4 mother?	4 su madre?
5 father?	5 su padre?
6 uncle (aunt)?	6 su tío (a)?
7 grandfather (grandmother)?	7 su abuelo (a)?
8 cousin?	8 un (a) primo (a)?
9 friend?	9 un (a) amigo (a)?
10 other relative?	10 otro pariente?

Are you . . .	Es . . .
1 single?	1 soltero (a)?
2 married?	2 casado (a)?
3 separated?	3 separado (a)?
4 divorced?	4 divorciado (a)?
5 widowed?	5 viudo (a)?
6 single, but living with your girlfriend (boyfriend)?	6 soltero (a), pero vive con su novia (o)?

Do you consider yourself to be . . .	Se considera . . .
1 homosexual?	1 homosexual?
2 bisexual?	2 bisexual?
3 heterosexual?	3 heterosexual?

Do you have any children?	Tiene *hijos*?
How many?	Cuántos?
What ages?	De qué *edades*?
Have you ever been married before?	Ha estado casado (a) *alguna vez*?
How many different sexual partners do you have in a month?	Cuántos amantes tiene por mes?
Do you have anal intercourse?	Practica coito anal?

Do you have . . .	Tiene . . .
1 primary education?	1 educación *primaria*?

2 secondary education?
3 college education?
4 graduate education?
5 professional education?
6 vocational education?

Is your religion . . .

1 Catholic?
2 Protestant?
3 Jewish?
4 Baptist?
5 Mormon?
6 Evangelist?
7 Episcopalian?
8 Christian Science?
9 Jehovah's Witness?
10 Muslim?
11 Buddhist?
12 Hindu?

2 educación *secundaria*?
3 educación *universitaria*?
4 estudios *graduados*?
5 educación *profesional*?
6 educación *vocacional*?

Su religión es . . .

1 Católica?
2 Protestante?
3 Judía?
4 Bautista?
5 Mormón?
6 Evangelista?
7 Episcopal?
8 Ciencia Cristiana?
9 Testigo de Jehová
10 Musulmán?
11 Budista?
12 Hindú?

3.2 OCCUPATIONAL HISTORY

Are you employed?
Do you work outside your home?
What type of work do (did) you do?

1 retired
2 teacher
3 secretary
4 housewife
5 salesperson
6 doctor
7 lawyer
8 engineer
9 student
10 architect

DATOS OCUPACIONALES

Tiene empleo?
Trabaja afuera de su casa?

En qué trabaja (trabajaba)?

1 jubilado (a)
2 maestro (a)
3 secretaria
4 ama de casa
5 vendedor (a)
6 médico (a) doctor (a)
7 abogado (a)
8 ingeniero (a)
9 estudiante
10 arquitecto (a)

11	accountant	11	contador (a)
12	farmer	12	campesino, agricultor
13	waiter (waitress)	13	camarero (a)
14	mechanic	14	mecánico (a)
15	factory worker	15	trabajador (a) de fábrica
16	truck driver	16	conductor (a) de camión
17	bus driver	17	conductor (a) de bus
18	taxi driver	18	conductor (a) de taxi
19	nurse	19	enfermero (a)
20	police officer	20	policia

Where do (did) you work?
How long have you worked there?
What was your first job?
What other jobs have you had?
How long did you work there?
Why did you change jobs?
Are you happy in your work?
Why?

En *dónde* trabaja (trabajaba)?
Hace *cuánto* tiempo que trabaja allí?
Cuál fue su *primer* empleo?
Qué otros empleos ha tenido?
Cuanto tiempo trabajó *allí*?
Por qué cambió de trabajo?
Está *contento* (a) en su trabajo?
Por qué?

Do (Did) you work with . . .

En su trabajo, está (estaba) expuesto (a) a . . .

1	lead?	1	plomo?
2	insecticides?	2	insecticidas?
3	chemicals?	3	substancias *químicas*?
4	paints?	4	pinturas?
5	plastics?	5	plásticos?
6	other synthetic materials?	6	otras substancias *sintéticas*?
7	drugs?	7	drogas?
8	dusts?	8	polvos?
9	animals?	9	animales?
10	birds?	10	pájaros?
11	radiation?	11	irradiación?

When?
For how long?
Do (Did) you use any
precautionary measures?
What?

Cuándo?
Por cuánto tiempo?
Toma (tomaba)
precauciones?
Cuáles?

3.3 HOBBIES AND SOCIAL ORGANIZATIONS

PASATIEMPOS Y ORGANIZACIONES SOCIALES

Do you enjoy . . .

Le gusta . . .

1 sports?
2 reading?
3 movies?
4 music?
5 theater?
6 painting?
7 photography?
8 gardening?
9 carpentry?

1 el deporte?
2 leer?
3 el cine?
4 la música?
5 el teatro?
6 la pintura?
7 la fotografía?
8 la jardinería?
9 la carpintería?

Do you play an instrument?
Do you belong to groups
of . . .

Toca un instrumento?
Pertenece a grupos de . . .

1 the church?
2 the school?
3 sports?

1 la iglesia?
2 la escuela?
3 deportes?

3.4 INSURANCE AND ECONOMIC INFORMATION

SEGUROS E INFORMACIÓN ECONÓMICA

Are you the sole financial
support of your family?
About how much money
do you earn a month?
Does anyone else in the
family work?

Es el *único* que sostiene a
su familia?
Más o menos, *cuánto* gana
mensualmente?
Hay alguien *más* en la
familia que trabaja?

Who?	Quién?
How much do they earn?	*Cuánto* ganan ellos?
Do you receive financial assistance from any . . .	Recibe *ayuda financiera* de . . .
1 other people?	1 alguna *otra* persona?
2 organizations?	2 alguna *organización*?
Do you have . . .	Tiene *seguros* . . .
1 life insurance?	1 de vida?
2 hospital insurance?	2 para el hospital?
3 accident insurance?	3 para accidentes?
4 Medicare?	4 de Medicare?
5 other social assistance?	5 de otra asistencia social?
6 other public assistance?	6 de otra asistencia pública?
Do you have an insurance card?	Tiene una tarjeta de seguro médico?
Please show it to me.	Por favor, muéstremela.
I am going to copy your insurance card.	Voy a copiar su tarjeta de seguro.
Do you have a primary care doctor?	Tiene un médico general?
Who is it?	Quién es?

3.5 PATIENT PRIVACY INFORMATION

INFORMACIÓN DE LA PRIVACIDAD DEL PACIENTE

I would like to protect your privacy for health information.	Deseo proteger su privacidad de la información médica.
I am obligated to do so by law.	Tengo un deber legal de hacerlo.
I have the right by law to release your protected health information for . . .	Tengo derecho por ley de compartir su información médica protegida por razones tales como . . .

1 treatment of medical problems including . . .

a doctors.

b nurses.

c other health care givers involved in your care.

2 payment, including . . .
a insurance companies.
b ambulance companies.

c medical bill preparation.

3 health care operations, including . . .
a clinical improvement.
b peer review.

c business management.

d accreditation and licensing.

4 appointment reminders.

I cannot release information about your drug or alcohol use or about HIV testing without . . .

1 your written permission.
2 a court order.

If it is an emergency medical situation, I may release this information.

1 tratamiento de problemas médicos incluyendo . . .
a comunicación con doctores.
b comunicación con enfermeras.
c comunicación con otros profesionales de la salud ayudando en su cuidado médico.

2 pago, incluyendo . . .
a compañías de seguro.
b compañías de ambulancia.
c preparación de la cuenta médica.

3 operaciones del cuidado médico incluyendo . . .
a mejoras clínicas.
b revisiones profesionales de grupo.
c administración de negocios.
d acreditación y licenciatura.

4 recordatorios de la cita.

No puedo compartir información sobre su uso de drogas, alcohol o pruebas para el SIDA, sin su . . .

1 autorización por escrito.
2 una orden de la corte.

Si es una emergencia médica puedo compartir esta información.

Federal law does not protect medical privacy about . . .

1 crimes committed here.
2 crimes threatened here.
3 suspected child abuse.
4 abuse to you.
5 public health risks.
6 adverse events reported to the Federal Drug Administration.

I can release private medical information . . .

1 to your employer if the care was requested by your employer,
2 to the military if you are in the military.
3 to Worker's Compensation if it is needed to determine a compensation benefit.

4 if I need to arrange an organ transplant for you or a donation of tissue or organ by you.

Please list the names of family, friends, others, and their relationship to you, with whom I may share your medical information.

Las Leyes Federales no protegen la información médica privada sobre . . .

1 crímenes cometidos aquí.
2 crímenes amenazados aquí.
3 sospecha de abuso de niños.
4 abuso a usted.
5 riesgos a la salud pública.
6 eventos adversos cuando es necesario reportalos a la Administración de Drogas y Alimentos.

Yo puedo divulgar su información privada . . .

1 a su empresa si fue ésta la que solicitó el cuidado médico.
2 a los Servicios de las Fuerzas Armadas, si usted es militar.
3 a la Agencia de Compensación de Trabajadores si es necesario para determinar su beneficio de compensación.

4 si es necesario planear un transplante para usted o si usted hace una donación de un órgano o tejido.

Por favor, escriba el nombre de los miembros de la familia, amigos u otros, con quien yo pueda divulgar su información médica

Person's Name	Relationship to Patient	Nombre de la Persona	Tipo de Relación
_____	_____	_____	_____
_____	_____	_____	_____
_____	_____	_____	_____

If you feel your privacy rights have been violated you may file a complaint in writing.

The address is _____.
Do you have any questions about your privacy for health information?
I will give you the name of someone who can speak with you in your own language.

If you do not have questions, I need you to sign HERE.

Do you have a living will?

Would you like to prepare one?

Do you need special assistance because of . . .

1 impaired vision.
2 impaired hearing.
3 other physical or mental disabilities.

Do you have an organ donation card?

Would you like to have one?

Si usted cree que sus derechos de privacidad han sido violados, usted puede quejarse por escrito.

La dirección es _____.
Tiene alguna pregunta sobre su privacidad de la información médica?
Le daré el nombre de una persona que puede hablar en su propio idioma.

Si no tiene más preguntas, necesito que firme AQUÍ.

Tiene un testamento en vida?

Quiere preparar uno?

Necesita asistencia especial porque . . .

1 no puede ver.
2 no puede oír bien.
3 tiene otras dificultades fisicas o mentales.

Tiene una tarjeta para donar órganos?

Le gustaría tener una?

Chapter 4
PAST MEDICAL HISTORY

This chapter covers the traditional information needed for a complete medical background. There are questions on immunizations, foreign travel, and illnesses that may have been acquired abroad.

4.1 PAST HEALTH, HOSPITALIZATIONS, AND ILLNESSES	ESTADO DE SALUD, HOSPITALIZACIONES Y ENFERMEDADES ANTERIORES
How has your health been up until now . . .	Hasta ahora, cómo ha estado su salud . . .
1 good?	1 buena?
2 fair?	2 regular?
3 poor?	3 mala?

Do you have your own doctor?	Tiene su propio médico?
What is his (her) . . .	Cuál es su . . .
1 name?	1 nombre?
2 address?	2 dirección?
3 telephone number?	3 número de teléfono?
4 email address?	4 dirección electrónica?
5 fax number?	5 número de fax?
When was the last time you went to his (her) office?	Cuándo fue la última vez que fue a la clínica de su médico?
What was the visit for?	Por qué consultó a su médico?
Have you ever been in the hospital?	Ha estado en el hospital?
When was it?	Cuándo?
Why were you there?	Por qué?
How long were you there?	Cuánto tiempo estuvo allí?
Which hospital was it?	En qué hospital?
What is the address?	Cuál es la dirección?
Have you ever had a blood transfusion?	Ha recibido alguna transfusión de sangre?
When was it?	Cuándo?
Have you ever had surgery?	Ha sido operado alguna vez?
Did you have any complications with the surgery?	Tuvo alguna complicación con la cirugía?
What type . . .	Qué tipo . . .
1 stroke?	1 derrame cerebral?
2 heart attack?	2 ataque del corazón?
3 blood clot in the . . .	3 coágulo . . .
a leg?	a de la pierna?
b lung?	b del pulmón?
Did they operate . . .	Le operaron . . .
1 on your tonsils?	1 las amígdalas?

2 on your appendix?
3 on your gallbladder?
4 on your large intestine?
5 on your small intestine?
6 on your uterus?
7 on your ovaries?
   a the right one?
   b the left one?
   c both?
8 on your prostate?
9 for a hernia . . .
   a inguinal?
   b umbilical?
10 for cataracts?
11 on your kidneys . . .
   a for stones?
   b for removal?
   c for transplant?

Have you ever had a blood transfusion?

Have you had . . .
1 chicken pox?
2 measles?
3 rubella?
4 mumps?
5 whooping cough?
6 scarlet fever?
7 rheumatic fever?
8 tuberculosis?
9 hepatitis . . .
   a A?
   b B?
   c C?

Have you been pregnant?
How many times?

2 la apéndice?
3 la vesícula?
4 el intestino grueso?
5 el intestino delgado?
6 la matriz?
7 los ovarios?
   a el derecho?
   b el izquierdo?
   c ambos?
8 la próstata?
9 una hernia . . .
   a inguinal?
   b umbilical?
10 cataratas?
11 los riñones . . .
   a por piedras?
   b para remover?
   c por un transplante?

Ha tenido alguna transfusión de sangre?

Ha tenido . . .
1 varicela?
2 sarampión?
3 rubeola?[1]
4 paperas?
5 tos ferina?
6 escarlatina?
7 fiebre reumática?
8 tuberculosis?
9 hepatitis . . .
   a A?
   b B?
   c C?

Ha estado embarazada?
Cuántas veces?

[1]The translation of rubella into Spanish is rubeola. This is not a copy error.

Have you had a cesarean?	Ha tenido una cesárea?
Have you had a miscarriage?	Ha tenido un aborto espontáneo?

4.2 IMMUNIZATIONS AND TRAVEL ABROAD

INMUNIZACIONES Y VIAJES EN EL EXTERIOR

Have you ever traveled outside this country?	Ha viajado fuera de este país?
When?	Cuándo?
Where?[2]	Dónde?[2]
Were you sick?	Se enfermó?
Did you see a doctor?	Le vio un médico?

Cuál fue . . .

What was . . .
1 the diagnosis?
2 the treatment?

1 el diagnóstico?
2 el tratamiento?

Have you had vaccinations for . . .
1 diphtheria?
2 whooping cough?
3 polio?
4 tetanus?
5 smallpox?
6 typhoid fever?
7 cholera?
8 BCG?
9 yellow fever?
10 rubella?
11 measles?
12 hepatitis A or B?
13 anthrax?

Le han puesto vacunas de . . .
1 difteria?
2 tos ferina?
3 polio?
4 tétano?
5 viruela?
6 fiebre tifoidea?
7 cólera?
8 BCG?
9 fiebre amarilla?
10 rubeola?
11 sarampión?
12 hepatitis A o B?
13 ántrax?

When were they?
When was your last chest x-ray?
Where was it taken?

Cuándo?
Cuándo le tomaron su última radiografía del pecho?
Dónde se la sacaron?

[2]See index of countries, page 186.

Were the results . . .	Los resultados fueron . . .
1 normal?	1 normales?
2 abnormal?	2 anormales?

Have you been tested for tuberculosis?	Ha recibido la prueba de tuberculina?
When?	Cuándo?
Who tested you?	Quién le hizo la prueba?

Were the results . . .	Los resultados fueron . . .
1 positive?	1 positivos?
2 negative?	2 negativos?

4.3   SOCIAL HABITS

HÁBITOS SOCIALES

| Do you ever have problems sleeping? | Duerme bien? |
| How is your appetite? | Cómo está su apetito? |

Do you smoke/Have you ever smoked . . .	Fuma/Alguna vez fumó . . .
1 cigarettes?	1 cigarrillos?
2 pipe?	2 pipa?
3 cigars?	3 cigarros?
4 chewing tobacco?	4 rapé?
5 marijuana?	5 marihuana?

How much do you smoke a day?	Cuánto fuma al día?
How long have you been smoking?	Hace cuánto tiempo qué fuma?
Have you ever tried to stop?	Ha tratado de dejar de fumar?
Would you like to stop?	Le gustaría dejar de hacerlo?

Do you use/Have you used . . .	Usa/Ha usado . . .
1 cocaine?	1 cocaína?
2 heroin?	2 heroína?
3 other illicit drugs?	3 otras drogas ilícitas?

How long have you used it?	Hace cuánto tiempo que la usa?
Have you ever tried to stop?	Ha tratado de dejar de usarla?
Would you like to stop?	Le gustaría dejar de usarla?
Have you ever shared needles?	Comparte o ha compartido agujas?
Have you ever shared needles with someone with . . .	Ha compartido agujas con alguien que sufre de . . .

1 hepatitis?
2 AIDS?

1 hepatitis?
2 SIDA?

Do you drink . . .

Bebe . . .

1 beer?
2 wine?
3 whiskey?
4 coffee?
5 tea?

1 cerveza?
2 vino?
3 whiskey?
4 café?
5 té?

How much each day . . .

Cuánto bebe al día . . .

1 glass?
2 bottle?
3 cup?

1 vaso?
2 botella?
3 taza?

Do you drink when you are . . .

Bebe cuando está . . .

1 alone?
2 sad?
3 depressed?
4 happy?
5 in a social situation only?

1 solo (a)?
2 triste?
3 deprimido (a)?
4 alegre?
5 en una reunión social solamente?

Do you think you have a drinking problem?	Cree que tiene problemas de alcoholismo?
Would you like help?[3]	Quiere ayuda?[3]

---

[3]See page 170 for further questions about alcohol use.

Do you use any drugs or
medicines?
Which ones?
Why do you use them?
How long have you used them?

Who gave them to you?

Toma alguna droga o
medicina?
Cuáles?
Por qué las usa?
Hace cuánto tiempo qué las
usa?
Quién se las dio?

4.4 PAST MEDICAL HISTORY OF THE FAMILY

ANTECEDENTES MÉDICOS FAMILIARES

Is your father (mother) living?
What did he (she) die from?
How old was he (she) when he
(she) died?
Have you or anyone in your
family had . . . [4]

Vive su padre (madre)?
De qué murió?
Cuántos años tenía al morir?

Ha tenido usted o alguien
en su familia . . . [4]

1 high blood pressure?
2 hyperlipidemia . . .
   a high cholesterol?
   b high triglycerides?
3 heart disease?

4 heart attack?
5 stroke?
6 varicose veins?
7 thrombophlebitis?
8 blood clots . . .
   a in the legs?
   b in the lungs?
9 arteriosclerosis?
10 obesity?
11 kidney disease?

12 diabetes?

1 presión alta?
2 hiperlipidemia . . .
   a colesterol elevado?
   b triglicéridos elevados?
3 enfermedad del
   corazón?
4 ataque del corazón?
5 derrame cerebral?
6 várices?
7 tromboflebitis?
8 coágulos . . .
   a de las piernas?
   b del pulmón?
9 arteriosclerosis?
10 obesidad?
11 enfermedad de los
    riñones?
12 diabetes?

[4]If the answer is "si", then ask: Quién? (Who?)
Cuándo? (When?)

13	osteoporosis?	13	osteoporosis?
14	cancer? What type?	14	cáncer? Qué tipo?
15	bronchitis?	15	bronquitis?
16	tuberculosis?	16	tuberculosis?
17	pneumonia?	17	neumonía?
18	bleeding tendencies?	18	tendencias a sangrar?
19	anemias . . .	19	anemias . . .
	a sickle cell?		a células falciformes?
	b thalassemia?		b talasemia?
	c iron deficiency?		c deficiencia de hierro?
20	convulsions?	20	convulsiones?
21	mental retardation?	21	retraso mental?
22	psychiatric problems?	22	problemas psiquiátricos?
23	emotional problems?	23	problemas emocionales?
24	glaucoma?	24	glaucoma?
25	congenital defects?	25	defectos congénitos?
26	venereal diseases . . .	26	enfermedades venéreas . . .
	a gonorrhea?		a gonorrea?
	b syphilis?		b sífilis?
	c herpes?		c herpes?
	d AIDS?		d SIDA?
27	allergies?	27	alergias?
28	trouble with anesthesia?	28	algún problema con la anestesia?
29	asthma	29	asma

Are you allergic to . . .   Tiene alergia a . . .

1	foods . . .	1	las comidas . . .
	a eggs?		a los huevos?
	b milk?		b la leche?
	c seafood?		c los mariscos?
2	medicines . . .	2	las medicinas . . .
	a aspirin?		a la aspirina?
	b penicillin?		b la penicilina?
	c sulfa drugs?		c medicina con sulfa?
3	iodine?	3	yodo?

4 contrast medium?
5 latex?
6 pollen?
7 dust?
8 animals . . .
  a dogs?
  b cats?
  c others?

What happens to you?
Do you get . . .
  a rash?
  b shortness of breath?
  c swelling?
Have there been any other diseases?
Which ones?
Is there anything else you would like to tell me?

4 medio de contraste?
5 látex?
6 el polen?
7 el polvo?
8 los animales . . .
  a los perros?
  b los gatos?
  c otros?

Qué le pasa?
Sufre de . . .
  a erupción?
  b falta de aire?
  c hinchazón?
Ha padecido de alguna otra enfermedad?
Cuáles?
Hay algo más que quiera decirme?

Chapter 5
CHIEF COMPLAINT OR REVIEW OF SYSTEMS

Chapter 5 begins with a section about pain. In those cases where a detailed analysis of pain and the accompanying circumstances is needed, this section should be consulted. All the organ system sections contain at least the basic questions related to pain. In this way, the interviewer does not always have to refer back to the first section to continue his (her) investigation.

The other questions found in Chapter 5 are necessary for a complete investigation of each organ system. The gastrointestinal system section includes a brief nutritional history. The reproductive system is divided into various subsections: past pregnancies and deliveries, venereal infections, breast examinations and pap smear, menstrual history, sexual function, and menopause.

5.1 PAIN	EL DOLOR
Do you have OR have you had pain?	Tiene O ha tenido dolor?
How long have (did) you had (have) it?	Cuánto tiempo hace (hacía) que lo tiene (tenía)?
Did it develop . . .	Se inició . . .
1 slowly?	1 lentamente?
2 suddenly?	2 de repente?
Is this (Was that) the first time that that you have (had) this type of pain?[1]	Es (Fue) la primera vez que siente este dolor?[1]
When was the first time?	Cuándo fue la primera vez?
How long does (did) the pain last each time?	Cuánto le dura (duraba) cuando le viene (venía)?
Is (Was) it . . .	Es (Era) un dolor . . .
1 severe?	1 severo?
2 mild?	2 leve?
3 moderate?	3 moderado?
4 intermittent?	4 intermitente?
5 constant?	5 constante?

[1]Whenever using the past tense, ask "cuándo?" (when?). This is important throughout this chapter.

6 sharp?
7 boring?
8 colicky?
9 shooting?
10 burning?
11 cramping?
12 pressurelike?

6 agudo?
7 penetrante?
8 cólico?
9 fulgurante?
10 quemante?
11 como un calambre?
12 opresivo?

Where is (was) the pain?
Show me with one finger.
Has (Did) the pain changed
(change) location?
Where did the pain begin?
Where does (did) it hurt . . .

Dónde le duele (dolía)?
Señáleme con un dedo.
Ha *cambiado* (cambió) de
lugar?
Dónde le empezó?
Dónde le duele (dolía) . . .

1 the most?
2 the least?

1 más?
2 menos?

Does (Did) the pain radiate?
From where to where?

Se *corre* (corría) el dolor?
Hacia *dónde*?

Do (Did) you have the
pain . . .

Tiene (Tenía) el dolor . . .

1 all the time?
2 in the morning?
3 in the afternoon?
4 at night?
5 before eating?
6 after eating?
7 while eating?
8 when it is (was) cold?

9 when it is (was) hot?

10 when it is (was) humid?

11 when you are (were) . . .

a upset?
b worried?

1 *todo* el tiempo?
2 por la mañana?
3 por la tarde?
4 por la noche?
5 *antes* de comer?
6 *después* de comer?
7 *mientras* come (comía)?
8 cuando hace (hacía)
frío?
9 cuando hace (hacía)
calor?
10 cuando hay (había)
humedad?
11 cuando está
(estaba) . . .
a molesto (a)?
b preocupado (a)?

12	when you exercise (exercised)?	12	cuando hace (hacía) *ejercicio*?
13	when you urinate (urinated) . . . a at the beginning? b the whole time? c at the end?	13	cuando *orina* (orinaba) . . . a al empezar? b durante *todo* el tiempo? c al terminar?
14	when you defecate (defecated)?	14	cuando evacúa o *defeca* (defecaba)?
15	when you have (had) sexual relations?	15	cuando tiene (tenía) *relaciones sexuales*?
16	when you swallow (swallowed) . . . a liquids? b solids? c both?	16	cuando *traga* (tragaba) . . . a líquidos? b sólidos? c ambos?
17	when you . . . a stand (stood)? b sit (sat) down? c lie (lay) down? d walk (walked)? e climb (climbed) stairs? f bend (bent) over?	17	cuando . . . a está (estaba) *de pie*? b *está* (*estaba*) sentado (a)? c *está* (*estaba*) acostado (a)? d camina (caminaba)? e *sube* (*subía*) escaleras? f se agacha (agachaba)?

Is (Was) there anything that makes (made) the pain . . .

Hay (Había) *algo* que . . .

1 better?
2 worse?

1 lo alivie (aliviara)?
2 lo aumente (aumentara)?

What is (was) it?
Is (Was) there anything else that accompanies (accompanied) the pain?
Does (Did) the pain go away when you rest (rested)?

Qué es (era)?
Hay (Había) otras *molestias* que acompañan (acompañaban) el dolor?
Se *alivia* (*aliviaba*) el dolor al descansar?

Do (Did) you awake at night from this pain?
Lo *despierta* (despertaba)?

Do (Did) you take anything for the pain?
Toma (*Tomaba*) algo para el dolor?

Does (Did) it help?
Lo *alivia* (*aliviaba*)?

Does (Did) it make it worse?
Lo *aumenta* (*aumentaba*)?

5.1.1 Inflammation and Infection
Inflamación e Infección

Do you have OR have you had . . .
Tiene O ha tenido . . .

1 swelling HERE?
2 redness HERE?
3 tenderness HERE?
4 a sensation of warmth HERE?
5 limitation of movement HERE?
6 stiffness HERE?
7 itching HERE?

1 hinchazón AQUÍ?
2 enrojecimiento AQUÍ?
3 dolor AQUÍ?
4 calor AQUÍ?
5 limitación de movimiento AQUÍ?
6 rigidez AQUÍ?
7 picazón AQUÍ?

Has pus drained from the wound?
Ha salido *pus* de la herida?

5.2 HEAD AND NECK
CABEZA Y CUELLO

Do you have OR have you had pain HERE?
Tiene O ha tenido dolor AQUÍ?

What is (was) the pain like?
Cómo es (era) el dolor?

How long have (did) you had (have) it?
Cuánto tiempo hace (hacía) que lo tiene (tenía)?

How long does (did) the pain last each time?
Cuánto le dura (duraba) cuando le viene (venía)?

How often do (did) you have the pain?
Con qué *frecuencia* lo tiene (tenía)?

Does (Did) the pain radiate? From where to where?
Se *corre* (corría) el dolor? *Hacia* dónde?

Is (Was) there anything that makes (made) the pain . . .
Hay (Había) *algo* que . . .

1	better?	1	lo alivie (aliviara)?
2	worse?	2	lo aumente (aumentara)?

What is (was) it?

Qué es (era)?

Have you ever been hit in the . . .

Se ha golpeado . . .

1	head?	1	la cabeza?
2	face?	2	la cara?
3	neck?	3	el cuello?
4	eyes?	4	los ojos?
5	ears?	5	los oídos?
6	nose?	6	la nariz?

Have you ever lost consciousness?

Ha perdido el conocimiento?

For how long?

For cuánto tiempo?

When?

Cuándo?

What happened?

Que le pasó?

Do you wear . . .

Usa . . .

1	glasses?	1	anteojos?
2	contact lenses . . .	2	lentes de contacto . . .
	a for distance?		a para ver de lejos?
	b for close-up?		b para ver de cerca?
	c for reading?		c para leer?
	d all the time?		d todo el tiempo?
	e since when?		e desde cuándo?

Do you have OR have you had . . .

Tiene O ha tenido . . .

1	frequent . . .	1	frecuentemente . . .
	a headaches?		a dolor de cabeza?
	b earaches?		b dolor del oído?
	c colds?		c catarros?
	d stuffed-up nose?		d la nariz tapada?
2	many nosebleeds?	2	sangrado por la nariz?
3	many ear infections*?	3	salida de pus por los oídos (pus coming from your ears)?
4	burning of your eyes?	4	ardor en los ojos?

5 itching of your eyes?
6 tearing of your eyes?
7 redness of your eyes?

8 blurred vision?
9 decreased hearing?
10 ringing in your ear?
11 trouble breathing through your nose?
12 pain . . .
  a in your forehead?
  b under your eyes?
13 gums that bleed easily?

14 dentures?
15 frequent sores . . .
  a on your tongue?
  b in your mouth?

When was the last time you had a . . .

1 vision test?
2 hearing test?

5.3 CARDIOVASCULAR-RESPIRATORY SYSTEM

Do you have OR have you had . . .
1 pain in your chest?

Where is (was) the pain?
What is (was) the pain like?
How long have (did) you had (have) it?
How long does (did) the pain last each time?
How often do (did) you have the pain?

5 picazón en los ojos?
6 lagrimeo de los ojos?
7 enrojecimiento de los ojos?

8 visión nublada?
9 falta de oír?
10 zumbido en el oído?
11 dificultad al respirar por la nariz?
12 dolor . . .
  a en la frente?
  b debajo de los ojos?
13 encías que sangran fácilmente?

14 dentaduras postizas?
15 úlceras frecuentes . . .
  a en la lengua?
  b en la boca?

Cuándo fue el último examen especial de . . .

1 la vista?
2 los oídos?

SISTEMAS CARDIOVASCULAR-RESPIRATORIO

Tiene O ha tenido . . .

1 dolor de pecho?

Dónde le duele (dolía)?
Cómo es (era) el dolor?
Cuánto tiempo hace que lo tiene (tuvo)?
Cuánto le dura (duraba) cuando le viene (venía)?
Con qué frecuencia lo tiene (tenía)?

Is it worse when you breath?   Es peor cuando respira?
When you inhale/exhale?   Cuando inhala/exhala?
Does (Did) the pain radiate?   Se corre (corría) el dolor?
From where to where?   *Hacia* dónde?
Is (Was) there anything   Hay (Había) *algo* que . . .
which makes (made) the
pain . . .
   a better?   a lo alivie (aliviara)?
   b worse?   b lo aumente
             (aumentara)?

What is (was) it?   *Qué* es (era)?

2   shortness of breath . . .   2   sensación de falta de aire?
   a while exercising?   a al hacer *ejercicio*?
   b at rest?   b al descansar?
   c when you are (were)   c cuando está (estaba)
      upset?   *molesto* (a)?
3   difficulty in breathing . . .   3   *dificultad* para
                        respirar . . .
   a sitting?   a sentado (a)?
   b standing?   b de pie?
   c lying down?   c acostado (a)?
   d exercising?   d al hacer *ejercicio*?
   e at rest?   e al descansar?
   f when you are (were)   f cuando está (estaba)
      upset?   *molesto* (a)?
4   night sweats?   4   sudores por la noche?
5   palpitations?   5   palpitaciones?
6   frequent colds . . .   6   catarros *frecuentes* . . .
   a in winter?   a en el invierno?
   b in spring?   b en la primavera?
   c in summer?   c en el verano?
   d in fall?   d en el otoño?
7   a cough?   7   tos?
   Is (Was) it a dry cough?   Es (Era) *seca*?
   Is (Was) it productive?   Es (Era) con *flema*?
   Is (Was) the phlegm . . .   Es (Era) la *flema* . . .
   a foamy?   a espumosa?
   b thick?   b espesa?

c foul-smelling?
d clear?
e of what color?
f abundant?
g a little bit?
h blood-streaked?

When do (did) you cough?
Do (Did) you have pain
when you cough (coughed)?
Do (Did) you breathe easier
after coughing?

Is (Was) there any position
that makes (made) it . . .

1 better?
2 worse?

Is (Was) the _____
accompanied by . . . [2]

1 fever?
2 chills?
3 sweating?
4 tingling sensation . . .
    a in the face?
    b in the lips?
    c in the extremities?
5 dizziness?
6 nausea?
7 vomiting?
8 loss of consciousness?

9 fainting?
10 numbness . . .
    a in the lips?
    b in the extemities?

c con *mal* olor?
d clara?
e de *qué* color?
f abundante?
g poca?
h con *manchas* de
sangre?

A *qué horas* tose (tosía)?
Le *duele* (*dolía*) al toser?

Respira (Respiraba) *mejor*
después de toser?

Hay (Había) *alguna* posición
que . . .

1 la *alivie* (*aliviara*)?
2 la *aumente* (*aumentara*)?

Se *acompaña* (*acompañaba*)
_____ de . . . [2]

1 fiebre?
2 escalofríos?
3 sudores?
4 hormigueo . . .
    a en la *cara*?
    b en los *labios*?
    c en las extremidades?
5 mareo?
6 náusea?
7 vómitos?
8 *pérdida* del
conocimiento?

9 desmayo?
10 adormecimiento . . .
    a de los *labios*?
    b de las *extremidades*?

[2]Whenever this question form is used, fill in the blank with any of the symptoms found previously.

11 pain?

How many pillows do you
sleep with?
Since when?
Have you ever noticed . . .

1 swelling in your . . .
   a feet?
   b hands?
2 bluish color of your . . .

   a lips?
   b feet?
   c hands?
3 coldness of your . . .

   a feet?
   b hands?

What type of regular exercise
do you do?

How many stairs (blocks) can
you climb (walk)
without getting . . .

1 short of breath?
2 pain in your . . .
   a legs?
   b chest?

Does the _____ go away
when you stop?

11 dolor?

con *cuántas* almohadas
duerme?
Desde cuándo?
Ha *notado* que . . .

1 se le hinchan . . .
   a los pies?
   b las manos?
2 se le ponen morados
   (as) . . .
   a los labios?
   b los pies?
   c las manos?
3 se le mantienen fríos
   (as) . . .
   a los pies?
   b las manos?

Que tipo de ejercicio hace
regularmente?

Cuántas escaleras (cuadras)
puede subir (andar) sin
tener . . .

1 una sensación de ahogo?
2 dolor . . .
   a de las piernas?
   b del corazón?

Se desaparece _____
cuando para?

5.4 GASTROINTESTINAL SYSTEM

Do you have OR have you had
pain in your abdomen?
Where is (was) the pain?
Show me with one finger

SISTEMA GASTROINTESTINAL

Tiene O ha tenido dolor en
el estómago (stomach)?
Dónde le duele (dolía)?
Señáleme con un dedo.

What is (was) the pain like?
How long have (did) you had (have) it?
How long does (did) the pain last each time?
How often do (did) you have the pain?
Does (Did) the pain radiate?
From where to where?
Is (Was) there anything that makes (made) the pain . . .

1 better?
2 worse?

What is (was) it?

Do you get . . .

1 indigestion from . . .
2 pain with . . .
  a alcohol?
  b spices?

  c coffee?
  d milk?
  e fats?

Do you have OR have you had problems . . .

1 swallowing?
2 chewing?

Do you often . . .

1 feel nauseated?
2 vomit?
3 burp?

When you vomit (vomited), is (was) it . . .

1 accompanied by nausea?

Cómo es (era) el dolor?
Cuánto tiempo hace (hacía) que lo tiene (tenía)?
Cuánto le dura (duraba) cuando le viene (venía)?
Con qué frecuencia lo tiene (tenía)?
Se corre (corría) el dolor?
Hacia dónde?
Hay (Había) algo que . . .

1 lo alivie (aliviara)?
2 lo aumente (aumentara)?

Qué es (era)?

Le causa . . .

1 indigestión . . .
2 dolor . . .
  a el alcohol?
  b la comida condimentada?
  c el café?
  d la leche?
  e las grasas?

Tiene O ha tenido problemas para . . .

1 tragar?
2 masticar?

Tiene frecuentemente . . .

1 náusea?
2 vómitos?
3 eructos?

Cuando vomita (vomitaba) es (era) . . .

1 acompañado de náusea?

2	before eating?	2	antes de comer?
3	while eating?	3	mientras come?
4	immediately after eating?	4	inmediatamente después de comer?
5	several hours after eating?	5	varias horas después de comer?
6	not related to when you eat (ate)?	6	sin relación con la comida?
7	in large quantities?	7	mucho?
8	in small quantities?	8	poco?
9	similar in composition to what you have just eaten?	9	parecido a lo que comió?
10	bloody?	10	con sangre?
11	green?	11	de color verde?
12	like coffee grounds?	12	de color café-negro (color of black coffee)?
13	acidic in taste?	13	de sabor ácido?
14	bitter in taste?	14	de sabor amargo?

Have you ever noticed . . .   Ha notado . . .

1	black stools?	1	heces negras?
2	mucus in the stools?	2	heces con moco?
3	bloody stools?	3	heces con sangre?
4	fatty stools?	4	heces con grasa?
5	foul-smelling stools?	5	heces con mal olor?
6	foamy stools?	6	heces espumosas?
7	clay-colored stools?	7	heces de color de arcilla?
8	a yellow color to your skin or eyes?	8	un color amarillo en la piel o en los ojos?
9	itching of your skin?	9	picazón en la piel?
10	a change in the color of your urine?	10	un cambio del color de la orina?
11	pain on defecation?	11	dolor al defecar?
12	anal itching?	12	picazón del ano?
13	blood on the toilet paper?	13	sangre en el papel higiénico?

Have you noticed any change in your bowel habits?

Defeca normalmente?

How often do you defecate?
When did you last defecate?

Cada cuánto defeca?
Cuándo defecó por última
vez?

Do you have OR have you
had . . .

Tiene O ha tenido . . .

1 constipation?
2 gas?
3 diarrhea?
4 urgency?
5 incontinence of stool?

1 estreñimiento?
2 gases?
3 diarrea?
4 urgencia para defecar?
5 incontinencia del heces?

Since when?
How many times a day do
(did) you have diarrhea?
How many times a night?

Desde cuándo?
Cuántas veces al dia
tiene (tenía) diarrea?
Cuántas veces en la noche?

Is (Was) it accompanied
by . . .
1 pain?
2 intestinal cramps?
3 straining?
4 gas?
5 fever?
6 chills?
7 nausea?
8 vomiting?
9 relief after defecating?

Se acompaña (acompañaba)
de . . .
1 dolor?
2 calambres intestinales?
3 pujo?
4 gases?
5 fiebre?
6 escalofríos?
7 náusea?
8 vómitos?
9 alivio al terminar de
defecar?

Is (Was) the diarrhea . . .

La diarrea es (era) . . .

1 of what color?
2 bloody?
3 with fat?
4 with mucus?
5 very foul-smelling?

1 de qué color?
2 con sangre?
3 con grasa?
4 con moco?
5 con muy mal olor?

When you finish (finished), do
(did) you feel as if you still
have (had) to defecate?

Al terminar, se queda
(quedaba) con deseos de
defecar?

5.4.1 *Nutritional History*

Do (Did) you have a good appetite?
How much do (did) you weigh?
What is the most/least you've weighed?

Do (Did) you eat . . .

1 more than usual?
2 less than usual?
3 the same as usual?

Are (Were) you on a diet?
Do (Did) you want to gain weight?
Do (Did) you want to maintain your present weight?
Do (Did) you want to lose weight?

Has your weight . . .

1 increased?
2 decreased?

Do you usually eat (drink) . . .

1 bread?
2 rice?
3 beans?
4 cereal?
5 macaroni?
6 green vegetables?
7 yellow vegetables?
8 fruits?
9 meats?
10 fish?
11 poultry?
12 sweets?
13 cheeses?

Historia de Nutrición

Tiene (Tenía) buen apetito?
Cuánto pesa (pesaba)?
Cuál fue su peso máximo/mínimo?

Come (Comía) . . .

1 más que lo usual?
2 menos que lo usual?
3 igual que siempre?

Está (Estaba) a dieta?
Quiere (Quería) subir de peso?
Quiere (Quería) mantener su peso actual?
Quiere (Quería) bajar de peso?

Su peso ha . . .

1 subido?
2 bajado?

Generalmente come (bebe) . . .

1 pan?
2 arroz?
3 frijoles?
4 cereal?
5 pastas?
6 vegetales verdes?
7 vegetales amarillos?
8 frutas?
9 carnes?
10 pescado?
11 aves?
12 dulces?
13 quesos?

14	milk?		14	leche?
15	eggs?		15	huevos?
16	butter?		16	mantequilla?
17	margarine?		17	margarina?

Is there anything you don't eat because . . .

Hay algo que no come porque . . .

1	you don't like it?		1	no le gusta?
2	it makes you feel bad?		2	le cae mal?
3	you are allergic to it?		3	tiene alergia?
4	it's against your religion?		4	está en contra de su religión?

How many times a day do you eat?
When?
Who prepares the food?

Cuántas veces al día come?
Cuándo?
Quién prepara la comida?

Is the food usually . . .

Es la comida normalmente . . .

1	raw?		1	cruda?
2	fried?		2	frita?
3	baked?		3	horneada?
4	broiled?		4	asada al fuego?
5	boiled?		5	hervida?
6	spicy?		6	picante?
7	greasy?		7	grasosa?
8	salty?		8	muy salada?

How much liquid do you drink a day?
More or less.
Do you use any sugar substitute?
Do you take vitamins?
Why?
Which ones?
Do you take herbal remedies?

Do you take calcium?

Qué cantidad de líquidos toma diariamente?
Más o menos.
Usa algún azúcar artificial?
Toma vitaminas?
Por qué?
Cuáles?
Toma algún remedio hierbal?
Toma calcio?

5.5 URINARY TRACT

Do you have OR have you had . . .

1 problems with your . . .
   a kidneys?
   b bladder?
2 pain from your . . .
   a kidneys?
   b bladder?

Where is (was) the pain?
What is (was) the pain like?
How long have (did) you had (have) it?
How long does (did) the pain last each time?
How often do (did) you have the pain?
Does (Did) the pain radiate?
From where to where?
Is (Was) there anything which makes (made) the pain . . .

1 better?
2 worse?
What is (was) it?
3 pain on urination . . .
   a at the start?
   b the whole time?

   c at the end?
4 burning on urination?
5 to urinate more frequently?
6 a feeling of urgency to urinate?
7 to urinate in larger quantities?

SISTEMA URINARIO

Tiene O ha tenido . . .

1 molestias de . . .
   a los riñones?
   b la vejiga?
2 dolor de . . .
   a los riñones?
   b la vejiga?

Dónde le duele (dolía)?
Cómo es (era) el dolor?
Cuánto tiempo hace (hacía) que lo tiene (tenía)?
Cuánto le dura (duraba) cuando le viene (venía)?
Con *qué frecuencia* lo tiene (tenía)?
Se *corre* (corría) el dolor?
Hacia dónde?
Hay (Había) *algo* que . . .

1 lo alivie (*aliviara*)?
2 lo aumente (*aumentara*)?
Qué es (era)?
3 dolor al *orinar* . . .
   a al empezar?
   b durante *todo* el tiempo que orina?
   c al terminar?
4 *ardor* al orinar?
5 que orinar con más *frecuencia*?
6 *urgencia* para orinar?
7 que orinar en *mayores* cantidades?

8 to urinate a lot at night?

9 difficulty starting the urinary stream?

10 an interrupted urinary stream?

11 a decrease in . . .
   a the size of the urinary stream?
   b the force of the urinary stream?

12 dribbling after urination?

13 stress incontinence?

14 small stones in your urine?

15 cloudy urine?

16 pink urine?

17 urine like Coca-Cola . . .

   a at the start?
   b in the middle?
   c at the end?

Is (Was) the _____ accompanied by . . . [3]

1 fever?
2 chills?
3 malaise?
4 low back pain?

Have you ever involuntarily dripped urine when you . . .

1 laugh?

8 que orinar *más* por la noche?

9 *dificultad* para empezar a orinar?

10 el chorro *interrumpido*?

11 disminución . . .
   a del grueso del chorro urinario?
   b de la fuerza del chorro urinario?

12 goteo al terminar de orinar?

13 incontinencia de esfuerzo?

14 orina con arenilla?

15 orina turbia?

16 orina rosada?

17 orina color de Coca-Cola . . .

   a al empezar?
   b en el medio?
   c al terminar?

Se acompaña (acompañaba) _____ con . . . [3]

1 fiebre?
2 escalofríos?
3 malestar general?
4 dolor de la espalda?

Orina por gotas involuntariamente cuando . . .

1 se ríe?

---

[3]Fill in the blank with any of the symptoms found previously.

2 sneeze?
3 cough?
4 run?
5 exercise?

Do you have to wear a
protective pad?

2 estomuda?
3 tose?
4 corre?
5 hace ejercicio?

Tiene que usar una toalla
protectiva?

5.6 REPRODUCTIVE SYSTEM

SISTEMA REPRODUCTIVO

Do you have OR have you had
pain HERE?
What is (was) the pain like?
How long have (did) you had
(have) it?
When was the last time?
How long does (did) the pain
last each time?
Does (Did) the pain radiate?
From where to where?

Is (Was) there anything which
makes (made) the pain . . .

1 better?
2 worse?

What is (was) it?

Tiene, O ha tenido dolor
AQUÍ?
Cómo es (era) el dolor?
Cuánto tiempo hace que lo
tiene (tenía)?
Cuándo fue la última vez?
Cuánto dura (duraba)
cuando le viene (venía)?
Se corre (corría) el dolor?
Hacia dónde?

Hay (había) algo que . . .

1 lo alivie (aliviara)?
2 lo aumente (aumentara)?

Qué es (era)?

5.6.1 History of Past Pregnancies and Deliveries

Historias de Partos y Embarazos Anteriores

How many times have you
been pregnant?
How many children do you
have?
Did you breast-feed them?

Have you ever had . . .

Cuántas veces ha estado
embarazada?
Cuántos hijos tiene?

Les dio el pecho?

Ha tenido . . .

1 babies that were . . .
  a large?
  b small?
  c premature?
  d congenitally malformed?

2 multiple births . . .

  a twins?
  b more than two?
3 a forceps delivery?
4 a cesarean?
5 a child that was born . . .

  a feet first?
  b with the cord around
    the neck?
6 a child that was dead?

7 a child that died shortly
  after birth?

8 problems with the
  placenta?
9 a postpartum hemorrhage?

10 a miscarriage?
11 an abortion?
12 with your pregnancy have
   you ever had . . .

   a diabetes?
   b high blood pressure?
   c leg swelling?

   d liver problems?

How many weeks pregnant
were you when you had . . .

1 niños . . .
  a grandes?
  b pequeños?
  c prematuros?
  d con defectos de
    nacimiento?

2 nacimientos
  múltiples . . .
  a gemelos (as)?
  b más de dos?
3 un parto con fórceps?
4 una cesárea?
5 un niño que haya
  nacido . . .
  a de pies?
  b con el cordón
    alrededor del cuello?
6 un niño que haya
  nacido muerto?
7 un niño que haya
  muerto poco después
  de nacer?
8 algún problema con la
  placenta?
9 una hemorragia
  después del parto?
10 un aborto espontáneo?
11 un aborto provocado?
12 con el embarazo ha
   tenido problemas
   con . . .

   a diabetes?
   b alta presión de sangre?
   c hinchazón de las
     piernas?
   d el hígado?

Cuántas semanas de
embarazo tenía cuando
tuvo . . .

1 the abortion?	1 el aborto provocado?
2 the miscarriage?	2 el aborto espontáneo?
How long was your labor with the . . .	Cuánto le duró el trabajo de parto con . . .
1 first child?	1 su primer niño?
2 other children?	2 sus otros niños?
How much did your children weigh?	Cuánto pesaron sus niños?

5.6.2 Venereal Infections

Infecciones Venéreas

Do you have OR have you had a genital infection?

Tiene O ha tenido alguna infección genital?

With the infection do (did) you have . . .

Se acompañaba (acompañaba) la infección con . . .

1 itching of you genitals?
2 burning of your genitals?
3 redness of you genitals?

1 picazón de los genitales?
2 ardor de los genitales?
3 enrojecimiento de los genitales?

4 inguinal swelling?
5 inguinal tenderness?
6 sores on your genitals?
7 pus from the sores?

4 hinchazón de la ingle?
5 dolor de la ingle?
6 úlceras en los genitales?
7 pus saliendo de las úlceras?

8 vaginal secretion?
9 fever?

8 flujo vaginal?
9 fiebre?

Have you ever had a test for . . .

Le han hecho una prueba para . . .

1 syphilis?
2 gonorrhea?
3 herpes?
4 human papilloma virus?
5 AIDS?

1 sifilis?
2 gonorrea?
3 herpes?
4 el virus de papiloma humana?
5 SIDA?

When?	Cuándo?
Were the results . . .	Los resultados fueron . . .
1 positive?	1 positivos?
2 negative?	2 negativos?
Where you treated?	Recibió tratamiento?
With what?	Con qué le trataron?

5.6.3 Breast Examination and Pap Smear

Examen del Seno y Papanicolaou

When was your last . . .	Cuándo fue su último . . .
1 breast examination?	1 examen del seno?
2 Pap smear?	2 Papanicolaou?
3 mammogram?	3 mamograma?
Were the results . . .	Los resultados fueron . . .
1 normal?	1 normales?
2 abnormal?	2 anormales?
Did you have a biopsy?	Tuvo una biopsia?
Have you noticed . . .	Ha notado . . .
1 a change in the . . .	1 algún cambio en . . .
a size of your breast (nipples)?	a el tamaño de los senos (los pezones)?
b shape of your breast (nipples)?	b la forma de los senos (los pezones)?
c consistency of your breasts (nipples)?	c la consistencia de los senos (los pezones)?
2 any secretion from the nipples?	2 alguna secreción de los pezones?
3 rash around your nipples?	3 una erupción de los pezones?
4 any pain or swelling . . .	4 hinchazón o dolor . . .
a of your breasts?	a de los senos?
b of your nipples?	b de los pezones?
c under your arms?	c debajo del brazo?

How many children do you have?
Did you breast-feed them?
Are you breast-feeding now?

Is your . . .

1   husband circumcised?
2   sexual partner circumcised?

Cuántos hijos tiene?

Les dio de mamar?
Está dando de mamar ahora?

Está circunciso . . .

1   su esposo?
2   la persona con quien tiene relaciones sexuales?

5.6.4 Menstrual History

How old were you when your period began?
Do you still have it now?

When was your . . .

1   last period?
2   second to last period?

Is your period usually . . .

1   regular?
2   early?
3   late?

How long does it last?

Do you have a . . .

1   light flow?
2   heavy flow?
3   clots . . .
    a small?
    b large?

How many . . .

1   pads do you use a day?

2   tampons?

Historia Menstrual

A qué edad le vino su regla por primera vez?
La tiene todavía?

Cuándo fue su . . .

1   última regla?
2   penúltima regla?

Su regla normalmente es . . .

1   puntual?
2   adelantada?
3   atrasada?

Cuánto tiempo le dura?

Sale . . .

1   poca sangre?
2   mucha sangre?
3   coágulos . . .
    a pequeños?
    b grandes?

Cuántos (as) . . .

1   toallas sanitarias usa cada día?

2   tampones?

How many days pass between periods?

Cada cuántos días le viene?

Do you bleed in between periods?

Sangra entre reglas?

With your period do you . . .

Con su regla tiene . . .

1 gain weight?
2 have severe cramps?
3 have breast tenderness?
4 have swelling of your . . .
  a hands?
  b feet?
  c breasts?
5 have back pain?
6 become . . .
  a depressed?
  b emotional?

1 aumenta de peso?
2 cólicos fuertes?
3 dolor de los senos?
4 hinchazón de . . .
  a las manos?
  b los pies?
  c los pechos?
5 dolor de espalda?
6 tendencia a . . .
  a deprimirse?
  b estar más sensible?

5.6.5 Sexual Function

Función Sexual

Do you have OR have you had any change in your desire to . . .

Tiene O ha tenido un cambio en su deseo de . . .

1 make love with . . .

  a a woman?
  b a man?
2 masturbate?

1 tener relaciones sexuales con . . .

  a una mujer?
  b un hombre?
2 masturbarse?

Do you have OR have you had any problems with . . .

Tiene O ha tenido problemas con . . .

1 erection? . . .
  a there is (was) none?
  b is (was) it difficult to achieve?
  c is (was) it painful?
2 ejaculation? . . .
  a there is (was) none?

1 la erección? . . .
  a no la tiene (tenía)?
  b le cuesta (costaba)?

  c es (era) dolorosa?
2 la eyaculación? . . .
  a no hay (había)?

b is (was) it difficult to
   achieve?
c is (was) it premature?
d is (was) it painful?
e is (was) it bloody?
3 orgasm? . . .
   a there is (was) none?
   b is (was) it difficult to
      achieve?
   c is (was) it painful?
4 the quantity of genital
   secretions? . . .

   a is (was) it excessive?
   b is (was) it too little?

Do you have OR have you had
pain during sexual relations
. . .

1 before intercourse?
2 during intercourse?
3 after intercourse?

Are you content with your
sexual relations?
Would you like to talk with a
sexual counselor?

b le cuesta (costaba)?

c es (era) prematura?
d es (era) dolorosa?
e es (era) con sangre?
3 el orgasmo? . . .
   a no hay (había)?
   b le cuesta (costaba)?

   c es (era) doloroso?
4 la cantidad de
   secreciones genitales?
   . . .
   a es (era) excesiva?
   b es (era) poca?

Tiene O ha tenido dolor
durante sus relaciones
sexuales . . .

1 antes del acto sexual?
2 durante el acto sexual?
3 después del acto sexual?

Está satisfecho (a) con sus
relaciones sexuales?
Quiere hablar con un
consejero sobre el sexo?

5.6.6 Menopause

Have you gone a year without
a period?

Have you noticed . . .

1 any changes in your
   periods?
2 hot flashes?

3 sweating?

La Menopausia

Ha pasado un año sin tener
la regla?

Ha notado . . .

1 algún cambio en su
   regla?
2 sensación de calor en
   la cara?
3 que suda mucho?

4	dryness of your skin?	4	sequedad de su piel?
5	a decrease in vaginal secretions?	5	disminución de las secreciones vaginales?
6	difficulty or pain with entrance of the penis?	6	dificultad o dolor al entrar el pene?
7	vaginal bleeding with intercourse?	7	sangre por la vagina con el acto sexual?
8	tiredness?	8	cansancio?
9	that you are . . . a depressed? b nervous? c irritable?	9	que está . . . a deprimida? b nerviosa? c irritable?
10	trouble sleeping?	10	problemas para dormir?
11	bone fractures?	11	fractura de los huesos?

You are going through menopause.

Está pasando por la menopausia.

This is normal for a woman of your age.

Es normal para una mujer de su edad.

Are the symptoms severe?

Los síntomas son muy fuertes?

The symptoms will pass by themselves.

Los síntomas pasarán por sí solos.

I can give you something to make you more comfortable.

Puedo darle algo para ayudarle.

5.7 ENDOCRINE SYSTEM

SISTEMA ENDÓCRINO

Do you have OR have you had pain HERE?

Tiene O ha tenido dolor AQUÍ?

What is (was) the pain like?

Cómo es (era) el dolor?

How long have (did) you had (have) it?

Cuánto tiempo hace que lo tiene (tenía)?

How long does (did) the pain last each time?

Cuánto dura (duraba) cuando le viene (venía)?

How often do (did) you have the pain?

Con qué frecuencia lo tiene (tenía)?

Does (Did) the pain radiate?
From where to where?

Se corre (corría) el dolor?
Hacía dónde?

Is (Was) there anything that
makes (made) the pain . . .

Hay (Había) algo que . . .

1 better?
2 worse?

1 lo alivie (aliviara)?
2 lo aumente (aumentara)?

What is (was) it?

Qué es (era)?

Have you OR has anyone else
noticed . . .

Ha notado O le han hecho
notar . . .

1 a big change in your
weight . . .
a an increase?
b a decrease?
2 any change in your
skin? . . .
a is it darker?
b is it a finer texture?
c is it a rougher texture?
3 any change in your
voice? . . .
a is it higher?
b is it lower?
4 any problem . . .
a concentrating?
b sleeping?
5 any change in your
breasts? . . .
a an increase in size?
b secretions?

1 un cambio grande en su
peso? . . .
a ha subido?
b ha bajado?
2 algún cambio en su
piel? . . .
a es más oscura?
b es más fina?
c es más áspera?
3 algún cambio en su
voz? . . .
a es más alta?
b es más baja?
4 algún problema en . . .
a concentrarse?
b dormir?
5 algún cambio en los
pechos? . . .
a han crecido?
b han salido
secreciones?

6 any change in the . . .
a quantity of your total
body hair?
b quantity of hair on your
head?
c color of your hair?

6 algún cambio en . . .
a la cantidad del pelo
del cuerpo?
b la cantidad del pelo
de la cabeza?
c el color del pelo?

d texture of your hair?
e distribution of your hair?

7 any change in your periods?
8 any change in your facial features?
9 any change in your desire for sexual relations?
10 an intolerance to . . .
   a the cold?
   b the heat?
11 that you are more tired?
12 that you are more nervous?
13 that you perspire more than usual . . .
   a during the day?
   b at night?
14 that you are more thirsty?
15 that you urinate more?
16 that you eat more?
17 that you eat more and do not gain weight?

When you were a child, did you ever have radiation to . . .
1 your head?
2 your neck?

Have you ever noticed a lump in your neck?

5.8 HEMATOLOGIC SYSTEM

Do you have OR have you had pain HERE?
What is (was) the pain like?

d la textura del pelo?
e la localización del pelo?

7 algún cambio en su regla?
8 algún cambio en su cara?
9 algún cambio en sus deseos sexuales?
10 que no aguanta . . .
   a el frio?
   b el calor?
11 que se cansa más?
12 que se pone más nervioso (a)?
13 que suda más que normal . . .
   a por el día?
   b por la noche?
14 que tiene más sed?
15 que orina más?
16 que come más?
17 que come más y no engorda?

De niño (a), recibió radiación en . . .
1 la cabeza?
2 el cuello?

Ha notado una masa en el cuello?

SISTEMA HEMATOLÓGICO

Tiene O ha tenido dolor AQUÍ?
Cómo es (era) el dolor?

How long have (did) you had (have) the pain?

Cuánto tiempo hace que lo tiene (tenía)?

How long does (did) the pain last each time?

Cuánto le dure (duraba) cuando le viene (venía)?

How often do (did) you have the pain?

Con qué frecuencia lo tiene (tenía)?

Does (Did) the pain radiate?

Se corre (corría) el dolor?

From where to where?

Hacía dónde?

Is (was) there anything that makes (made) the pain . . .

Hay (Había) algo que . . .

1 better?
2 worse?

1 lo alivie (aliviara)?
2 lo aumente (aumentara)?

What is (was) it?

Qué es (era)?

What is your blood type?

Qué tipo de sangre tiene?

Do (Did) you bruise easily?

Se le hacen (hacían) moretones sin causa aparente?

Do (did) you bleed . . .
1 easily from . . .
   a your nose?
   b your gums?
2 a lot from a cut?
3 for a long time?

Sangra (Sangraba) . . .
1 fácilmente de . . .
   a la nariz?
   b las encías?
2 mucho de una herida?
3 por mucho tiempo?

5.9 MUSCULO-SKELETAL SYSTEM

SISTEMA MÚSCULO-ESQUELÉTICO

Which hand do you use most . . .

Que mano utiliza más . . .

1 the right?
2 the left?
3 both the same?

1 la derecha?
2 la izquierda?
3 igual las dos?

Do you have OR have you had . . .

Tiene 0 ha tenido . . .

1 any broken bones?

1 fracturas?

2 to wear a brace of any type?
3 muscle weakness?
4 trouble . . .

a climbing stairs?
b getting up from a chair?
5 muscle spasms?
6 pain in your . . .
a bones?
b muscles?
c neck?
d shoulders?
e elbows?
f wrist?
g fingers?
h hips?
i knees?
j ankles?
k toes?
l back?

Where is (was) the pain?
What is (was) the pain like?
How long have (did) you had (have) it?
How long does (did) the pain last each time?
Does (Did) the pain radiate?
From where to where?
Is (Was) there anything that makes (made) the pain . . .

1 better?
2 worse?

What is (was) it?

Do you have pain . . .

1 at night?
2 in the morning?

2 que llevar corsé?
3 debilidad muscular?
4 dificultad en las piernas para . . .

a subir escaleras?
b levantarse de una silla?
5 calambres musculares?
6 dolor en . . .
a los huesos?
b los músculos?
c el cuello?
d los hombros?
e los codos?
f las muñecas?
g los dedos?
h las caderas?
i las rodillas?
j los tobillos?
k los dedos grandes?
l la espalda?

Dónde le duele (dolía)?
Cómo es (era) el dolor?
Cuánto tiempo hace que lo tiene (tenía)?
Cuánto le dura (duraba) cuando le viene (venía)?
Se corre (corría) el dolor?
Hacia dónde?
Hay (Había) algo que . . .

1 lo alivie (aliviara)?
2 lo aumente (aumentara)?

Qué es (era)?

Tiene dolor . . .

1 por la noche?
2 por la mañana?

3	with motion?	3	cuando se mueve?
4	at rest?	4	cuando descansa?

Is the pain associated with . . .   El dolor está acompañado por . . .

1	swelling?	1	hinchazón?
2	redness?	2	enrojecimiento?
3	sensation of warmth?	3	calor?
4	limitation of movement?	4	limitación de movimiento?
5	stiffness?	5	rigidez?

5.10 NERVOUS SYSTEM

5.10.1 Cranial Nerves

Do you have OR have you had . . .

SISTEMA NERVIOSO

Nervios Craneales

Tiene O ha tenido . . .

1	trouble smelling?	1	dificultad para sentir los olores?
2	a sensation of . . .	2	sensación de olores . . .
	a odd odors?		a raros?
	b unpleasant odors?		b desagradables?
3	blindness?	3	ceguera?
4	blind spots?	4	manchas negras frente a los ojos?
5	blurred vision?	5	vista nublada?
6	double vision?	6	visión doble?
7	spots before your eyes?	7	manchas enfrente de los ojos?
8	pain behind your eyes?	8	dolor en los ojos?
9	trouble distinguishing colors?	9	dificultad para distinguir colores?
10	decreased sensation in your face?	10	pérdida de la sensibilidad en la cara?
11	trouble chewing?	11	dificultad para masticar?
12	trouble whistling?	12	dificultad para silbar?

13 trouble . . .	13 dificultad para . . .
a opening your eyes?	a abrir los ojos?
b closing your eyes?	b cerrar los ojos?
14 decreased taste sensation?	14 *dificultad* para sentir los sabores?
15 taste sensations that are . . .	15 *sensación* de sabores . . .
a odd?	a raros?
b unpleasant?	b desagradables?
16 loss of hearing?	16 *pérdida* del oído?
17 difficulty in hearing?	17 *dificultad* para oír?
18 the sensation that noises are louder?	18 la *sensación* de que los sonidos son más fuertes?
19 ringing in your ears?	19 *zumbido* en los oídos?
20 trouble swallowing?	20 *dificultad* para tragar?
Since when?[4]	Desde *cuándo*?[4]
Where?	Dónde?
Did it develop . . .	Se inició . . .
1 slowly?	1 lentamente?
2 suddenly?	2 de repente?
Has it gotten . . .	La *molestia* ha . . .
1 better?	1 mejorado?
2 worse?	2 empeorado?

5.10.2 Sensory

Sensibilidad

Do you have OR have you had . . .	Tiene O ha tenido . . .
1 loss of tactile sensation?	1 *falta* de sensibilidad táctil?
2 trouble distinguishing . . .	2 *dificultad* para distinguir . . .

[4]The following four questions are to investigate any symptoms found in motor and coordination, sensory and cranial nerves.

a heat on your skin?	a el *calor* en la piel?
b cold on your skin?	b el *frío* en la piel?
3 tingling sensations?	3 hormigueos?
4 numbness?	4 adormecimiento?

5.10.3 Motor and Coordination

Movilidad y Coordinación

Do you have OR have you had . . .

Tiene O ha tenido . . .

1 loss of coordination?

1 *pérdida* de coordinación?

2 loss of balance?

2 *pérdida* del equilíbrio?

3 dizziness? . . .
a Did you spin around?
b Did the objects spin around?

3 mareo? . . .
a Daba usted *vueltas*?
b Le daban *vueltas* los objetos?

5.10.4 Special

Especial

Do you have OR have you had . . .

Tiene O ha tenido . . .

1 loss of . . .

a rectal control?
b bladder control?
2 trouble speaking clearly?
3 trouble understanding what you are asked?
4 loss of memory for . . .

a recent events?
b past events?
5 trouble . . .
a reading?
b writing?
6 loss of consciousness?

1 *pérdida* del control para . . .

a defecar?
b orinar?
2 *dificultad* para hablar?
3 *dificultad* para entender lo que le preguntan?
4 problemas para *recordar* . . .

a hechos *recientes*?
b hechos pasados?
5 *problemas* para . . .
a leer?
b escribir?
6 *pérdida* del conocimiento?

5.10.5 Convulsions and Headaches

Convulsiones y Dolores de Cabeza

Have you ever been hit in the head?

Alguna vez le golpearon la cabeza?

Do you have OR have you had convulsions?

Tiene O ha tenido convulsiones?

When did you have your . . .

Cuándo tuvo . . .

1 first convulsion?
2 last convulsion?

1 la primera convulsion?
2 la última convulsión?

How often do (did) you have them?

Con qué frecuencia le vienen (venían)?

Are (Were) the convulsions preceded by . . .

Están (Estaban) precedidas por . . .

1 a special odor?
2 a vision?
3 a constant thought?
4 a strange feeling?
5 any pain?

1 un olor especial?
2 una visión?
3 un pensamiento fijo?
4 una sensación rara?
5 algún dolor?

With the convulsions do (did) you . . .

Con las convulsiones . . .

1 lose consciousness?

1 pierde (perdía) el conocimiento?

2 bite your tongue?

2 se muerde (mordía) la lengua?

How long does (did) each convulsion last?

Cuánto le dura (duraba) cada convulsíon?

After a convulsion, how long are (were) you . . .

Después de una convulsíon, cuánto tiempo . . .

1 unconscious?

1 está (estaba) inconciente?

2 disoriented?

2 está (estaba) desorientado (a)?

Do (Did) you take medicine
for the convulsions?

Recibe (Recibía)
tratamiento?

What kind?
For how long?

Qué tipo?
Por *cuánto* tiempo?

Are the convulsions . . .

Ahora, las convulsiones
han . . .

1 better now?
2 worse now?

1 mejorado?
2 empeorado?

Do you have OR have you
had headaches?

Tiene O ha tenido *dolor* de
cabeza?

Are (Were) they . . .

Son (Eran) . . .

1 mild?
2 moderate?
3 severe?

1 leves?
2 moderados?
3 fuertes?

Where is (was) the pain?
Does (Did) it radiate?
From where to where?
What is (was) the pain like?
How long does (did) the
pain last each time?
How often do (did) you
have the pain?
In what year did you first
have the pain?
When was the last time?

Dónde le duele (dolía)?
Se *corre* (corría) el dolor?
Hacia dónde?
Cómo es (era) el dolor?
Cuánto le dura (duraba)
cuando le viene (venía)?
Con qué *frecuencia* lo
tiene (tenía)?
En que año tuvo el dolor
por primera vez?
Cuándo fue la última vez?

Is (Was) there anything that
makes (made) the pain . . .

Hay (Había) *algo* que . . .

1 better?
2 worse?

2 lo alivie (aliviara)?
2 lo aumente (aumentara)?

What is (was) it?

Qué es (era)?

Is (Was) the pain preceded
by . . .

Está (Estaba) el dolor
precedido por . . .

1 a special odor?

1 un olor *especial?*

2 a vision?	2 una visión?
3 a constant thought?	3 un pensamiento *fijo*?
4 a strange feeling?	4 una sensación *rara*?
5 nausea?	5 náusea?
6 vomiting?	6 vómitos?

Is (Was) the pain accompanied by other problems: What?
Are the headaches . . .

Siente (Sentía) otras *molestias* con el dolor? Cuáles?
Ahora, los dolores han . . .

1 better now?	2 mejorado?
2 worse now?	2 empeorado?

Chapter 6
INSTRUCTIONS FOR THE PHYSICAL EXAMINATION

This chapter begins with the general instructions needed for the physical examination. These particular phrases are repeated only in those organ-system sections where they form a large part of the patient's instructions.

As in Chapter 5, each organ system has its own section. With the exception of the nervous system, each section contains complete instructions for the physical examination of that particular system. For the examination of cranial nerves II, III, IV, VI, VIII, and IX, the examiner should refer to section 6.2, *Head and Neck.* The other phrases in this chapter are self-explanatory. However, there are a few points to keep in mind. When the instructions are linguistically complicated, as in the examination of the ocular fundus, the instructions are divided into single phrases. The examiner must remember to employ all the expressions needed to communicate the entire instruction.

Example:

Please . . .	Por favor . . .
1 focus HERE.	1 mire AQUÍ.
2 don't move your eyes.	2 *no* mueva los ojos.
3 don't move your head.	3 *no* mueva la cabeza.
4 don't blink.	4 *no* parpadee.
5 look into the light.	5 *mire* la luz.

The sections for the urinary tract and the endocrine system are short because of the use of laboratory examinations for diagnosis. There are no instructions for the physical examination of the hematologic system, since this examination is almost exclusively based on observation and laboratory tests.

6.1 GENERAL INSTRUCTIONS	**INSTRUCCIONES GENERALES**
I am going to examine you.	Voy a *examinarle.*
Please undress except for your underwear.	Por favor desvístase *menos* su ropa interior.
Please undress completely.	Por favor, desvístase completamente.
Please put this gown on with the opening in the . . .	Por favor, póngase la bota con la abertura . . .
1 front.	1 en frente.
2 back.	2 atrás.
Please . . .	Por favor . . .
1 lie down.	1 acuéstese.

2	sit down.	2	siéntese.	
3	stand up.	3	levántese.	
4	bend over forward.	4	dóblese hacia delante.	
5	bend over backward.	5	dóblese hacia atrás.	
6	lean forward.	6	inclínese hacia delante.	
7	lean backward.	7	inclínese hacia atrás.	
8	lie on your . . .	8	acuéstese . . .	
	a right side.		a sobre el lado derecho.	
	b left side.		b sobre el lado izquierdo.	
	c stomach.		c boca abajo.	
	d back.		d boca arriba.	
9	bend your knees.	9	doble las rodillas.	
10	turn your head . . .	10	mueva la cabeza . . .	
	a to the right.		a a la derecha.	
	b to the left.		b a la izquierda.	
11	bend your head.	11	doble la cabeza.	
12	turn over.	12	dése vuelta.	
13	don't talk.	13	no hable.	
14	lie still.	14	quédese quieto (a).	

Please do THIS.
Relax.
Are your comfortable?
THIS won't hurt.
Does THIS hurt?
Can you feel IT?
I'm sorry if THIS makes you uncomfortable.
It will only take a moment longer.
That's enough.
Once more.
Very good.
Thank you.
You may get dressed now.
I will talk with you when you are finished.

Por favor, haga ESTO.
Cálmese.
Está cómodo (a)?
ESTO no le dolerá.
Le duele ESTO?
Puede sentirLO?
Lo siento si ESTO le molesta.
Solo un momento más.

Suficiente.
Otra vez.
Muy bien.
Gracias.
Puede vestirse.
Hablaré con usted cuando termine.

6.2 HEAD AND NECK

EXAMEN FÍSICO DE LA CABEZA Y EL CUELLO

I am going to examine your . . .

Voy a *examinarle* . . .

1	head.	1	la cabeza.
2	eyes.	2	los ojos.
3	ears.	3	los oídos.
4	nose.	4	la nariz.
5	mouth.	5	la boca.
6	throat.	6	la garganta.
7	neck.	7	el cuello.

Do you have pain when I bend your neck?

Tiene *dolor* cuando le doblo el cuello?

Please swallow.

Por favor *trague.*

Again.

Otra vez.

Please . . .

Por favor . . .

1 read THIS.

1 lea ESTO.

2 how many fingers do you see?

2 *cuántos* dedos ve?

3 follow my finger with your eyes.

3 *siga* mi dedo con los ojos.

4 don't move your head.

4 no *mueva* la cabeza.

5 cover your *eye* like THIS.

5 tápese el ojo ASÍ.

6 where do you see my finger?

6 *dónde* ve mi dedo?

7 focus HERE.

7 mire AQUÍ.

8 don't move your eyes.

8 *no* mueva los ojos.

9 don't blink.

9 *no* parpadee.

10 look into the light.

10 *mire* la luz.

11 open your eyes.

11 *abra* los ojos.

12 close your eyes.

12 *cierre* los ojos.

13 look . . .

13 *mire* . . .

a up.

a arriba.

b down.

b abajo.

c to the side.

c *al lado.*

d HERE.

d AQUÍ.

I will touch your *eye* with
THIS.
Don't be afraid.

Please tell me . . .

1 when you . . .
   a can hear THIS.
   b cannot hear THIS.
   c can feel THIS.
   d cannot feel THIS.
2 if THIS is . . .
   a louder in one ear.
   b softer in one ear.
   c equal in both ears.

Breathe through your nose.

Please . . .

1 open your mouth wider.
2 stick out your tongue.
3 say "ah."
4 move your tongue from
   side to side.
5 lift up your tongue.

6.3 CARDIOVASCULAR-
RESPIRATORY
SYSTEMS

I am going to . . .

1 examine your lungs.

2 examine your heart.
3 take your pulse.
4 take your blood pressure.

Please . . .

1 sit down
2 lean forward.

Voy a tocar el ojo con
ESTO.
No tenga miedo.

Por favor *dígame* . . .

1 cuando . . .
   a pueda oir ESTO.
   b no pueda oir ESTO.
   c pueda sentir ESTO.
   d no pueda sentir ESTO.
2 si ESTO es . . .
   a *más* fuerte en un oído.
   b *más* suave en un oído.
   c *igual* en ambos oídos.

Respire por la nariz.

Por favor . . .

1 *abra* la boca más.
2 *saque* la lengua.
3 diga "*ah.*"
4 mueva la lengua de *lado*
   a *lado.*
5 *levante* la lengua.

EXAMEN FÍSICO DE
LOS SISTEMAS
CARDIOVASCULAR-
RESPIRATORIO

Voy a . . .

1 examinarle los
   pulmones.
2 examinarle el *corazón.*
3 tomarle el *pulso.*
4 tomarle la *presión.*

Por favor . . .

1 siéntese.
2 inclínese hacia

				adelante.
3	lie down.		3	acuéstese.
4	lie on your . . .		4	*acuéstese* sobre . . .
	a right side.			a su lado *derecho.*
	b left side.			b su lado *izquierdo.*
5	stand up.		5	levántese.
6	don't talk.		6	*no* hable.
7	breathe deeply through		7	respire *profundo* con la
	your mouth, . . . again.			boca abierta, . . . otra
				vez.
8	inspire.		8	inspire.
9	hold it.		9	*no* saque el aire.
10	exhale.		10	exhale.
11	take a deep breath.		11	respire *profundo.*
12	relax.		12	descanse.
13	breathe normally.		13	respire *normalmente.*
14	cough.		14	tosa.
15	say "33."		15	diga "*treinta y tres.*"
16	say "e."		16	diga "*e.*"
17	climb THESE stairs.		17	suba ESTAS escaleras.
18	walk on THIS.		18	camine sobre ESTO.

Do you feel dizzy?

Se siente *mareado* (a)?

6.4 GASTRO-INTESTINAL SYSTEM

EXAMEN FÍSICO DEL SISTEMA GASTRO-INTESTINAL

I am going to examine your . . .
1 abdomen*.
2 rectum.

Voy a examinar su . . .
1 estómago (stomach).
2 ano.

Please . . .

1 try and relax.
2 don't cross your legs.
3 inflate your stomach.
4 suck in your stomach.
5 take a deep breath.

Por favor . . .

1 cálmese.
2 *no* cruce las piernas.
3 *infle* el estómago.
4 *meta* el estómago.
5 inspire *fuerte.*

6 hold it.
7 relax.
8 cough.
9 lie on your . . .
    a right side.
    b left side.
10 bend your leg.
11 straighten out your
    other leg.

Please do it again.

6 *no saque el aire.*
7 *descanse.*
8 *tosa.*
9 *acuéstese sobre su
    lado . . .*
    a derecho.
    b izquierdo.
10 doble la pierna.
11 estire la otra pierna.

Por favor, otra vez.

6.5 URINARY TRACT

I am going to examine your
kidneys.

Please . . .

1 sit up.
2 lean forward.
3 remove your underwear.

Does THIS hurt?

EXAMEN FÍSICO DEL SISTEMA URINARIO

Voy a examinarle los
riñones.

Por favor . . .

1 siéntese.
2 inclínese hacia adelante.
3 quítese la ropa interior.

Le duele ESTO?

6.6 REPRODUCTIVE SYSTEM

I am going to examine . . .
1 your breasts.
2 your pelvis.
3 your penis.
4 your testicles.
5 for hernia.
6 your genitals.

Do you know how to
examine your breasts?

EXAMEN FÍSICO DEL SISTEMA REPRODUCTIVO

Le voy a examinar . . .
1 los senos.
2 la pelvis.
3 el pene.
4 los testículos.
5 si tiene hernias.
6 los genitales.

Sabe cómo examinarse sus
senos?

How often do you do it?
It is important that you
examine your breasts every
____ weeks (months).
Would you like to learn
how?

Con qué *frecuencia* lo hace?
Es *importante* que usted se
examine los senos cada
____ semanas (meses).
Le gustaría *aprender* cómo
hacerlo?

Please . . .

Por favor . . .

1 remove your
  underwear.
2 stand up.
3 cough.
4 bear down.
5 slide closer to the edge
  of the table.
6 put your legs up HERE.

1 *quítese* su ropa interior.

2 levántese.
3 tosa.
4 puje.
5 *acérquese* al borde de
  la mesa.
6 ponga las piernas
  AQUÍ.

7 open your legs more.
8 relax your muscles.
9 calm yourself.
10 put your arms like
   THIS.

7 *abra* más las piernas.
8 *relaje* los músculos.
9 cálmese.
10 ponga los brazos ASÍ.

6.7 ENDOCRINE SYSTEM

EXAMEN FÍSICO DEL SISTEMA ENDÓCRINO

Please swallow.
Again.

Trague, por favor.
Otra *vez*.

6.8 MUSCULO-SKELETAL SYSTEM

EXAMEN FÍSICO DEL SISTEMA, MÚSCULO-ESQUELÉTICO

Please . . .

Por favor . . .

1 push against my hand as
  hard as you can.
2 squeeze my fingers as
  hard as you can.

1 *empuje* fuerte mi mano.

2 *apriete* fuerte mis dedos.

3 don't let me move your . . .	3 *no* me deje mover su . . .
a head.	a cabeza.
b arm.	b brazo.
c leg.	c pierna.
4 raise your . . .	4 levante . . .
a arm.	a el brazo.
b leg.	b la pierna.
5 relax and let me move your . . .	5 *relájese* y déjeme moverle . . .
a arm.	a el brazo.
b leg.	b la pierna.
6 repeat THIS same motion.	6 repita ESTE mismo movimiento.

6.9 NERVOUS SYSTEM

EXAMEN FÍSICO DEL SISTEMA NERVIOSO

6.9.1 Mental Status Examination[1]

Examen del Estado Mental[1]

What is your name?	Cómo se *llama*?
How old are you?	*Cuántos* años tiene?
When were you born?	En qué fecha nació?
Where are you?	Qué lugar es *éste*?
Why are you here?	*Por qué* está aquí?
Who am I?	Quién soy?

What . . .	Qué . . .
1 day is this?	1 día es hoy?
2 month is this?	2 mes es *éste*?
3 year is this?	3 año es *éste*?

How much is _____ times _____?	*Cuánto* es _____ por _____?

What did you eat for breakfast?	*Qué* desayunó?

Who is the President of the United States?	*Quién* es el presidente de los Estado Unidos?

---

[1]For additional questions on memory and recall see page 156.

6.9.2 Cranial Nerves[2]

Does THIS smell like . . .
1 cinnamon?
2 clove?
3 mint?
4 alcohol?
5 tobacco?

Don't let me open your . . .
1 mouth.
2 eyes.

Please . . .
1 smile.
2 whistle.
3 try to close your eyes.
4 shrug your shoulders.
5 don't let me move your head.
6 stick our your tongue.
7 move it from side to side.

6.9.3 Sensory

Close your eyes.
Tell me when you feel SOMETHING.
Where do you feel IT?

Please tell me if THIS is . . .
1 hot.
2 cold.
3 like a prick.
4 like a tap.
5 moving . . .
   a upward.
   b downward.

Nervious Craneales[2]

Huele ESTO a . . .
1 canela?
2 clavo?
3 menta?
4 alcohol?
5 tabaco?

No me deje abrir . . .
1 su boca.
2 sus ojos.

Por favor . . .
1 sonría.
2 silbe.
3 *intente* cerrar los ojos.
4 levánte sus hombros.
5 *no* me deje mover su cabeza.
6 saque le lengua.
7 *muévala* de lado a lado.

Sensibilidad

Cierre los *ojos.*
Dígame cuando sienta ALGO.
Dónde LO siente?

Siente ESTO . . .
1 caliente.
2 frío.
3 como un *pinchazo.*
4 como un *toquecito.*
5 moviéndose . . .
   a hacia arriba.
   b hacia abajo.

[2]For cranial nerves II, III, IV, VI, VIII, and IX see *Head and Neck* (p. 68).

6.9.4 Motor

Please . . .

1 relax.
2 relax your . . .
  a arm.
  b leg.
  c foot.
  d wrist.
3 put your hands like THIS.
4 pull as hard as you can.

Movilidad

Por favor . . .

1 cálmese.
2 relaje . . .
  a el brazo.
  b la pierna.
  c el pie.
  d la muñeca.
3 ponga las manos ASÍ.
4 haga *fuerza*.

6.9.5 Coordination

Please . . .

1 close your eyes.
2 keep them shut.
3 stand up with your feet together.
4 hold your arms out straight.
5 walk heel to toe (LIKE THIS).
6 touch my finger with your finger and then touch your nose.
7 put your heel on your ankle.
8 run your heel up and down your leg.

DO IT faster.
Do IT with the other . . .

1 hand
2 leg.

Coordinación

Por favor . . .

1 *cierre* los ojos.
2 manténgalos *cerrados*.
3 párese con los pies *juntos*.
4 extienda sus brazos *al frente*.
5 camine con un pie delante del otro (ASÍ).
6 *toque* mi dedo con su dedo y luego toque su nariz.
7 *tóquese* el tobillo con el talón.
8 *deslize* el talón sobre su pierna.

HágaLO más rápido.
HágaLO con la otra . . .

1 mano.
2 pierna.

Chapter 7
GENERAL TREATMENT, TESTING AND FOLLOW-UP

Chapter 7 begins with a section on general treatment. These are patient instructions that do not deal with medications.

Example:

You need to . . .	Necesita . . .
1 stay in bed.	1 reposar en cama.
2 avoid excess work.	2 evitar trabajar *demasiado*.
3 take a vacation.	3 ir de vacaciones.

Section 7.2 contains a list of common laboratory examinations. They are grouped in subsections according to organ systems. Page 184 also contains an index of commonly requested tests in alphabetical order. In Section 7.3 the technical names of the specialists are given in English. The Spanish translation gives a simplified explanation of each specialty. The literal translation of the Spanish explanation is given in parentheses. Remember that an asterisk* indicates when this free translating is used.

Example:
You need to see . . .

1   a cardiologist*.

Necesita ver un . . .

1   especialista en enfermedades del corazón (the heart).

7.1   GENERAL TREATMENT

You have a problem with your ____.[1]
I don't know what the problem is.

I want you to see a ____ specialist.

You need to . . .

1   have more tests.
2   be hospitalized . . .
     a immediately.
     b in the near future.
3   stay in bed.
4   relax.
5   sleep . . .
     a more.
     b less.

TERAPIA GENERAL

Tiene un *problema* con ____.[1]
No sé que es *lo que* le molesta.

Quiero que le *vea* un especialista en enfermedades de ____.

Necesita . . .

1   *más* pruebas.
2   hospitalizarse . . .
     a inmediatamente.
     b próximamente.
3   *reposar* en cama.
4   descansar.
5   dormir . . .
     a más.
     b menos.

[1]Throughout this chapter, fill in the blank with the appropriate words.

6	avoid getting . . .	6	evitar . . .
	a upset.		a molestarse.
	b overtired.		b cansarse.
7	get . . .	7	hacer . . .
	a more exercise.		a *más* ejercicios.
	b less exercise.		b *menos* ejercicios.
8	avoid excess work.	8	evitar trabajar *demasiado.*
9	change jobs to one . . .	9	cambiar a un trabajo . . .
	a more active.		a *más* activo.
	b less active.		b *menos* activo.
10	take a vacation.	10	ir de *vacaciones.*
11	enjoy yourself more.	11	divertirse más.
12	live in a . . .	12	vivir en un clima . . .
	a drier climate.		a *más* seco.
	b more humid climate.		b *más* húmedo.
	c cooler climate.		c *más* frío.
	d warmer climate.		d *más* caliente.
13	eat . . .	13	comer . . .
	a more ____.		a más ____.
	b less ____.		b menos ____.
14	drink . . .	14	beber . . .
	a more ____.		a más ____.
	b less ____.		b menos ____.
15	never . . .	15	no . . .
	a eat ____.		a comer ____.
	b drink ____.		b beber ____.
16	maintain your weight.	16	*mantener* su peso.
17	try to . . .	17	tratar de . . .
	a gain ____ pounds.		a subir ____ libras.
	b lose ____ pounds.		b bajar ____ libras.
	c stop smoking.		c no fumar más.
	d stop drinking alcohol.		d no beber alcohol.
	e stop using drugs.		e no usar drogas.
18	avoid using your ____.	18	*evitar* uso de ____.
19	exercise your ____.	19	*hacer* ejercicio con ____.
20	practice THIS.	20	practicar ESTO.

21 keep your feet elevated . . .	21 mantener los pies elevados . . .
a all the time.	a *todo* el tiempo.
b when you rest.	b cuando descansa.
22 avoid straining when you defecate.	22 *evitar* esfuerzos cuando defeca.
23 avoid contact with ____.	23 evitar contacto con ____.
24 a cast on your ____.	24 un yeso en su ____.
25 have a blood transfusion.	25 una transfusión de sangre.
26 have an operation . . .	26 una operación . . .
a immediately.	a inmediatamente.
b in the near future.	b próximamente.

Don't get THIS wet.
You can continue your sexual
activites.
I need your permission to do
THIS procedure.
Please sign THIS permission
sheet.
I want to see you in ____.
Your next appointment is
____.
Please see the . . .
1 nurse.
2 receptionist.
3 secretary.

No se mojo ESTO.
Puede continuar sus
actividades sexuales.
Necesito su permiso para
hacer ESTE tratamiento.
Por favor, firme ESTA hoja
de autorización.
Quiero verle en ____.
Su próxima cita es ____.
Por favor, véase con la . . .
1 enfermera.
2 recepcionista.
3 secretaria.

7.1.1 General Test Instructions

*Instrucciones Generales
sobre las Pruebas*

This test is done as . . .

Esta prueba se hace como
. . .

1 an inpatient.

1 paciente dentro del
hospital.

2 an oupatient.

2 paciente fuera del
hospital.

The test will not hurt.	La prueba no le dolerá.
The test may cause some discomfort.	La prueba podría causar un poco de dolor.
They will keep you comfortable during the test.	Ellos lo harán sentirse cómodo durante la prueba.
You will receive sedation for the test.	Recibirá medicina para tranquilizarse durante la prueba.
You will not receive sedation for the test.	No recibirá medicina para tranquilizarse durante la prueba.
You need someone to drive you home.	Necesita a una persona que lo (la) lleve a su casa.
You will be able to drive yourself home.	Puede regresar a su casa solo (a).
Please stop THESE medicines ____ days before your . . .	Por favor, deje de tomar ESTAS medicinas ____ días antes de su . . .
1 test.	1 prueba.
2 surgery.	2 cirugía.
Do not eat or drink anything after midnight.	No coma ni beba nada después de la media-noche.
Do not drink or eat for ____ hours before the test.	No coma ni beba nada ____ horas antes de la prueba.
Drink ____ glasses of water before the test.	Tome ____ vasos de agua antes de la prueba.
Take all your medicine before the test.	Tome todas sus medicinas antes de la prueba.
Take only THESE medicines before the test.	Tome solamente ESTAS medicinas antes de la prueba.
Take no medicine before your test.	No tome ninguna medicina antes de la prueba.
Are you claustrophobic?	Sufre de claustrofobia?
You will have dye injected into your vein for the test.	Le van a inyectar una tinta dentro de su vena durante la prueba.

The dye will make you feel warm.	La tinta lo(a) hará sentir caliente.
Are you allergic to . . .	Es alérgico a . . .
1 iodine?	1 yodo?
2 x-ray dye?	2 materia de contraste para rayos-x?
3 shellfish?	3 mariscos?
You will have to drink something during the test.	Usted tiene que beber algo durante la prueba.

7.2 LABORATORY EXAMINATIONS[2]

7.2.1 Head and Neck

You need a . . .

1
  a vision test.
  b hearing test.
  c test for glaucoma.
2
  a throat culture.
  b nose culture.
  c ear culture.
3 test for allergies
4
  a head x-ray.
  b neck x-ray.
  c sinus x-ray.
5 CAT scan of your . . .

  a head.
  b sinus.

EXAMENES DEL LABORATORIO[2]

Cabeza y Cuello

Necesita . . .

1 un examen . . .
  a de la vista.
  b de los oídos.
  c para glaucoma.
2 un cultivo . . .
  a de la garganta.
  b de la nariz.
  c del oído.
3 una prueba para alergias.
4 una radiografía . . .
  a de la cabeza.
  b del cuello.
  c del seno.
5 una tomografía computada . . .
  a de la cabeza.
  b del seno.

---

[2]See Index of Commonly Requested Tests on page 184 for additional tests.

7.2.2 Cardiovascular-Respiratory System

You need . . .

1 an EKG.
2 an arteriogram.
3 a cardiac catherization.

4 a cardioversion.
5 a chest x-ray.

6 a sinus x-ray.
7 an echocardiogram.

8 a test for . . .
   a cholesterol.
   b triglycerides.
   c exercise tolerance.

   d pulmonary functions

9 a blood test.
10 bronchoscopy . . .
   a with biopsy.
11 a lung scan.

12 a CAT scan of your chest.

13 a PET scan.

Sistema Cardiovascular-Respiratorio

Necesita . . .

1 un electrocardiograma.
2 un arteriograma.
3 un cateterismo
   cardiaco.
4 una cardioversión.
5 una radiografía del
   pecho.
6 una radiografía del seno.
7 un ecocardiograma.

8 un examen de . . .
   a colesterol.
   b triglicéridos.
   c tolerancia al
     ejercicio.
   d las funciones
     pulmonares.
9 una prueba de sangre.
10 una broncoscopio . . .
   a con una biopsia.
11 un centellograma de
   los pulmones.
12 una tomografía
   computada del pecho.
13 una tomografía por
   emisión de positrones.

7.2.3 Gastrointestinal System

You need . . .

1 an upper GI series

2 a barium swallow.
3 an endoscopy.

Sistema Gastrointestinal

Necesita . . .

1 una serie
   gastrointestinal
   superior.
2 un trago de bario.
3 una endoscopia.

4 a barium enema.	4 un enema de bario.
5 a colonoscopy.	5 una colonoscopia.
6 to have . . .	6 un examen . . .
a a proctoscopy.	a proctoscopico.
b sigmoidoscopy.	b sigmoidoscopico.
c a urine analysis.	c de la orina.
d a stool analysis.	d de las heces.
e a liver function test.	e de la función hepática.
7 a liver biopsy.	7 una biopsia del hígado.
8 a stool culture.	8 un cultivo de heces.
9 a liver scan.	9 un centellograma del hígado.
10 a blood test.	10 una prueba de sangre.
11 an x-ray of ____.	11 una radiografia de ____.
12 a biopsy of ____.	12 una biopsia de ____.
13 a CAT scan.	13 una tomografía computada.
14 an ultrasound.	14 un examen de ondas ultrasónicas.
15 a cholangiogram . . .	15 un colangiograma . . .
a endoscopic.	a endoscopico.
b intravenous.	b intravenoso.
16 endoscopic retrograde cholangiopancreatography. (ERCP)	16 colangiopancreatografía retrograda endoscópica.
17 endoscopic ultrasound . . .	17 ultrasonido endoscópico
a with biopsy.	a con biopsia.

7.2.4 *Urinary Tract System*

You need . . .

1 a pyleogram . . .
   a intravenous (IVP).
   b retrograde.
   c excretory.

Sistema Urinario

Necesita . . .

1 un pielograma . . .
   a intravenoso.
   b retrógrado.
   c excretor.

2 a cystoscopy.	2 una cistoscopía.
3 to have a . . .	3 un análisis de . . .
a urine analysis.	a la orina.
b renal function test.	b la función de los riñones.
c blood tests.	c la sangre.
d urine culture.	d un cultivo de orina.
e 24-hour urine collection.	e una colección de orina durante veinticuatro horas.
4 a biopsy of . . .	4 una biopsia . . .
a the kidney.	a del riñón.
b the prostate.	b de la próstata.
5 an x-ray of your _____.	5 una radiografía de _____.
6 an ultrasound.	6 una ultrasonografía.
7 a catheter . . .	7 un catéter . . .
a Foley.	a Foley.
b Tenkckoff.	b Tenkckoff.
8 dialysis . . .	8 diálisis . . .
a hemo.	a hemo.
b peritoneal.	b peritoneal.
9 a prostate exam.	9 un examen de la próstata.

7.2.5 Reproductive System

You need . . .

1 to have . . .
   a a breast examination.
   b a pelvic examination.
   c a blood test.
2 to have . . .
   a a breast biopsy.
   b a uterine biopsy.
   c a cervical biopsy.
3 a colposcopy.
4 a culture . . .
   a of your vaginal secretions.

Sistema Reproductivo

Necesita . . .

1 un examen de . . .
   a los senos.
   b la pelvis.
   c la sangre.
2 una biopsia . . .
   a de los senos.
   b del útero.
   c del cervix.
3 una colposcopia.
4 un cultivo . . .
   a de las secreciones vaginales.

b for *Candida*.
c for *Trichomonas*.
d for Gonorrhea.
e for Syphilis.
f for Herpes.
g for Chlamydiae.
5 a mammogram.
6 a pap smear.
7 a rectal examination.
8 a semen analysis.
9 a pregnancy test.
10 a laparoscopy.
11 to have . . .
a an x-ray of your ____.

b a CAT scan.

c an MRI.

12 a pelvic ultrasound.

13 to have surgery . . .

a immediately.
b in the near future.

14 a blood test for HIV.

b para *Cándida*.
c para *Trichomonas*.
d para Gonorrea.
e para Sífilis.
f para Herpes.
g para Chlamydiae.
5 una mamografía.
6 un papanicolau.
7 un tacto *rectal*.
8 un análisis del semen.
9 una prueba para el
embarazo.
10 una laparoscopia.
11 tener . . .
a una radiografia de

____.
b una tomografia
computada
c una imagen por
resonancia
magnética.
12 un ultrasonido de la
pelvis.
13 tener una operación
. . .
a inmediatamente.
b en el futuro
próximo.
14 una prueba de sangre
para VIH.

7.2.6 *Endocrine System*

You need . . .

1 an analysis of . . .

a pituitary function.
b thyroid function.
c parathyroid function.
d pancreatic function.

Sistema Endocrino

Necesita . . .

1 un análisis de la función
. . .
a de la pituitaria.
b de la tiroides.
c del paratiroides.
d del páncreas.

e adrenal function.
f ovarian function.
g testicular function.
2 a glucose tolerance test.

3 an x-ray of your _____.
4 a blood test.
5 a urine analysis.
6 a CAT scan of _____.

7 an ultrasound of _____.

e de los adrenales.
f de los ovarios.
g de los testículos.
2 un examen de tolerancia
a la glucosa.
3 una radiografía de _____.
4 una prueba de sangre.
5 un análisis de la orina.
6 una tomografia
computada de _____.
7 un examen de ondas
ultrasónicas de _____.

7.2.7 Hematologic System

You need . . .

1 a complete blood count.

2 a bone marrow biopsy.

3 to have . . .
a a serum iron analysis.
b a blood clotting test.

c an analysis of your blood
type.
d a urine analysis.
e a stool analysis.
4 a transfusion of . . .
a blood.
b platelets.

Sistema Hematológico

Necesita . . .

1 un recuento de glóbulos
blancos y rojos.
2 una biopsia de la medula
ósea.
3 un *análisis* . . .
a del hierro en la sangre.
b de la coagulación de
la sangre.
c del tipo de sangre.

d de la orina.
e de las heces.
4 una transfusión . . .
a de sangre.
b de plaquetas.

7.2.8 Musculoskeletal System

You Need . . .

1 an x-ray of _____.

Sistema Músculo-
Esquelético

Necesita . . .

1 una radiografía de

_____.

2   a blood test.
3   a urine analysis.
4   to have a . . .
    a bone biopsy.
    b a muscle biopsy.
5   a muscle function test.

6   a joint . . .
    a aspiration.
    b injection.

7   an arthroscopy.
8   a cast.
9   a CAT scan.

10 an MRI.

2   una prueba de sangre.
3   un análisis de la orina.
4   una biopsia de . . .
    a los huesos.
    b los músculos.
5   un examen de la
    función muscular.
6   una . . .
    a punción articular.
    b inyección
      interarticular.
7   una artroscopia.
8   un yeso.
9   una tomografía
    computada.
10 una imagen por
    resonancia magnética.

7.2.9   Nervous System

You Need . . .

1   an x-ray of your . . .
    a head.
    b neck.
2   an EEG.
3   a brain scan.

4   a cerebral arteriogram.

5   a lumbar puncture.
6   a myelogram.
7   a CAT scan.

8   an MRI scan.

9   an audiogram.
10 a PET scan.

11 an echocardiogram.

Sistema Nervioso

Necesita . . .

1   una radiografía . . .
    a de la cabeza.
    b del cuello.
2   un electroencefalograma.
3   un centellograma del
    cerebro.
4   un arteriograma
    cerebral.
5   una punción lumbar.
6   un mielograma.
7   una tomografía
    computada.
8   una imagen por
    resonancia magnética.
9   un audiograma.
10 una tomografía por
    emisión de positrones.
11 un ecocardiograma.

7.3 SPECIALISTS*

You need to see . . .

1 a specialist in . . .

a internal medicine.
b otolaryngology.

c ophthalmology.
d cardiology.
e pulmonology.

f gastroenterology.

g hepatology.
h nephrology.

i urology.

j gynecology.
k obstetrics.

l endocrinology.

m orthopedics.

n hematology.
o neurology.
p dermatology.
q oncology.
r radiology.
s geriatrics.
t psychiatry.

u psychology.

ESPECIALISTAS*

Necesita ver a un . . .

1 especialista en
enfermedades de . . .
(specialist in diseases of)
a los órganos internos.
b los oídos, la nariz, la
garganta (ears, nose,
throat).
c los ojos (eyes).
d el corazón (the heart).
e los pulmones (the
lungs).
f el aparato digestivo
(the GI tract).
g el hígado (the liver).
h los riñones (the
kidneys).
i el aparato urinario
(urinary tract).
j la mujer (women).
k embarazos y partos
(pregnancy and
delivery).
l las hormonas (the
hormones).
m los huesos (the
bones).
n la sangre (the blood).
o los nervios (nerves).
p la piel (skin).
q cáncer (cancer).
r radiografías (x-rays).
s los ancianos (elders).
t problemas emocionales
(emotional problems).
u psicología.

v pediatrics.

w dental problems.

x nutrition.

y surgery.

v los niños (children).

w los dientes (the teeth).

x dietas y nutrición (diet and nutrition).

y cirugía.

Chapter 8
MEDICAL THERAPY AND PATIENT INSTRUCTIONS

Chapter 8 is devoted to medical therapy and patient instructions about the use of medications. There are two sections. Section 8.1, Instructions about Medicines, has six subsections that contain the vocabulary needed to explain how medicines should be taken, when they should be taken, and how much should be taken. There are phrases covering previous use of medications, instructions about prescriptions, and a list of possible side effects that patients may experience. The section also contains a series of instructions about the storage of medications.

Section 8.1.6 covers special instructions for the symptoms of insulin overdose and insufficiency. These instructions are written in two forms: the first to communicate directly with the patient and the second to explain the symptoms to family members.

Section 8.2 is an index of some seventy therapeutic and pharmacological classes of medications. It is not a list of medicines by generic or trade name. This information is presented so that the health worker may explain to his patient what type of medicine he or she is taking and why he is taking it.

The different therapeutic and pharmacological groups are listed alphabetically in English by their technical names. The Spanish translation is an explanation of what the medicine is designed to do.

Example:

I am going to treat you with . .	Le voy a tratar con . . .
1 an antiarrhythmic agent.	1 una medicina que mejora el ritmo de su corazón (a medicine that improves the rhythm of your heart).

In certain instances, more than just the category of medicine is given. This is done so that the health worker can give more complete information to his patient and still present a simple and understandable explanation.

Example:

I am going to treat you with . . .	Voy a tratar con . . .

1 insulin that is . . .
  a short-acting.
  b medium-acting.
  c long-acting.
	1 *insulina de acción* . . .
	  a corta.
	  b mediana.
	  c larga.

For those health workers who wish to give the specific name of a medication to their patient it is best simply to give the name in English. The patient will probably understand since the names are similar in English and in Spanish. (This is more true for the generic names than for the trade names).

8.1 INSTRUCTIONS ABOUT MEDICINES

8.1.1 Prescription Instructions

THIS is a prescription for your medicine.
You can have it filled at any drugstore.
You can renew it _____ times.
It is enough for . . .

1 _____ week(s).
2 _____ month(s).
3 _____ year(s).

Please call me . . .

1 when you need more.
2 if you do not feel better in _____.
3 If you feel worse.
4 if you have any questions.

If you have any reactions, stop the medicine at once and call me.

8.1.2 Past Use of Medicines

Have you ever taken THIS medicine before?
When?
For what?
How much did you take a day?

INSTRUCCIONES SOBRE LAS MEDICINAS

Instrucciones Sobre las Recetas

ÉSTA es una receta para su medicina.
La puede comprar en _cualquier_ farmacia.
Puede usar la receta _____ veces.
Es suficiente para . . .

1 _____ semana(s).
2 _____ mes(es).
3 _____ año(s).

Por favor, llámeme . . .

1 cuando necesite más.
2 si no se siente _mejor_ dentro de _____.
3 si se siente peor.
4 si tiene alguna _pregunta._

Si tiene cualquier molestia, deje de tomar la medicina inmediatamente y llámeme.

Empleo Anterior de Medicinas

Ha tomado ESTA medicina antes?
Cuándo?
Para qué?
Qué cantidad tomó diariamente?

For how long?
Did it help?
Did you have any reactions
to it?

Por cuánto tiempo?
Le alivió?
Tuvo alguna molestia?

8.1.3 How and When to Use the Medicine

Cómo y Cuándo Usar las Medicinas

I am going to give
you an injection.

Voy a ponerle una
inyección.

Take _____

Tome _____

1 pills every _____ hours.
2 teaspoons of syrup every
   _____ hours.
3 tablespoons of syrup
   every _____ hours.

1 píldoras cada _____ horas.
2 cucharaditas de jarabe
   cada _____ horas.
3 cucharadas de jarabe
   cada _____ horas.

Take them for _____

Tómelas por _____

1 days.
2 weeks.
3 months.

1 días.
2 semanas.
3 meses.

Please take the medicine . . .

Por favor, tome la
medicina . . .

1 _____ times a day.
2 before meals.
3 with meals.
4 after meals.
5 before bedtime.
6 before you exercise.

7 when you have _____.[1]
8 only when you really
   need it, because it may
   be habit-forming.

1 _____ veces al día.
2 antes de la comida.
3 con la comida.
4 después de la comida.
5 antes de acostarse.
6 antes de hacer
   ejercicios.
7 cuando tenga _____.[1]
8 solamente cuando la
   necesite mucho porque
   produce hábito.

[1]Fill in the blank with the appropriate symptom.

Drops	*Gotas*
Put ____ drops in . . .	Ponga ____ gotas en . . .
1 your nose.	1 la nariz.
2 your mouth.	2 la boca.
3 one eye (both eyes).	3 un ojo (ambos ojos).
4 one ear (both ears).	4 un oído (ambos oídos).

Cream	*Crema*
Apply the cream to the affected area.	Aplique la crema en el área afectado.

Applicators	*Aplicadores*
Squeeze the cream into the applicator and insert into the vagina.	Ponga la crema dentro del aplicador, e introdúzcalo dentro de la vagina.

Hormone Patch	*Parche de Hormona*
Apply the patch to the skin of your outer arms, buttocks, upper torso, or abdomen.	Aplique el parche en la superficie de la piel de la parte exterior de los brazos, glúteos, la parte superior del torso, o en el abdomen.

Suppository	*Supositorio*
Place the suppository in . . .	Meta el supositorio dentro de . . .
1 the rectum.	1 el recto.
2 the vagina.	2 la vagina.

Spray	*Spray*
Inhale the spray through your . . .	Inhale el spray por . . .

1 nose.
2 mouth.

Lozenge

Let it dissolve in your
mouth.
Let it dissolve under your
tongue.
Chew the tablet.

Powder

Mix _____
    teaspoons of powder
    with _____ cups of
    water.
    tablespoons of powder
    with _____ cups of
    water.

Drink it.
Gargle with the mixture.

Soak your _____ with the
mixture for _____ minutes.

Injection

1 subcutaneous
2 intramuscular

8.1.4 Common Side Effects

With THIS medicine you
may . . .

    1 be irritable.
    2 be depressed.

1 la nariz.
2 la boca.

Tableta

Deje que se *disuelva* en la
boca.
Deje que se disuelva *debajo*
de la lengua.
Mastique la tableta.

Polvo

Mezcle _____
    cucharaditas de polvo
    con _____ tazas de
    agua.
    cucharadas de polvo
    con _____ tazas de
    agua.

Tómela.
Haga gárgaras con la
mezcla.
Sumerja su _____ en la
mezcla por _____ minutos.

Inyección

1 subcutánea
2 intramuscular

Efectos Colaterales Comunes

Con ESTA medicina puede
tener . . .

    1 irritabilidad.
    2 depresión.

3	be agitated.	3	agitación.
4	have insomnia.	4	insomnio.
5	be dizzy.	5	mareos.
6	feel weak.	6	debilidad.
7	have blurred vision.	7	vista nublada.
8	have double vision.	8	visión doble.
9	have ringing in your ears.	9	zumbido de oídos.
10	note a bad taste in your mouth.	10	un sabor desagradable en la boca.
11	have a dry mouth.	11	sequedad de la boca.
12	be nauseated.	12	nausea.
13	be thirsty.	13	sed.
14	be hungry.	14	hambre.
15	lose your appetite.	15	falta de apetito.
16	have excess salivation.	16	salivación excesiva.
17	have diarrhea.	17	diarrea.
18	be constipated.	18	estreñimiento.
19	have a change in the color of your urine.	19	cambio de color de la orina.
20	have a different-smelling urine.	20	un olor especial de la orina.
21	have more vaginal secretions.	21	más flujo vaginal.
22	have palpitations.	22	palpitaciones.
23	have a rash.	23	una erupción.
24	have red spots.	24	manchas rojas.
25	cough.	25	tos.

8.1.5 Storage Instructions

Cómo Guardar las Medicinas

Keep THIS medicine . . .

Guarde ESTA medicina . . .

1 at room temperature.
2 in the refrigerator (not in the freezer).
3 out of strong light.
4 in a dry place.

1 a temperatura *ambiente*.
2 en el refrigerador (no en el congelador).
3 donde no haya mucha luz.
4 en un lugar seco.

5 away from heat.
6 away from children.

5 *fuera* del calor.
6 *fuera* del alcance de los niños.

8.1.6 Instructions for the Diabetic and Family

Instrucciones para el Diabético y la Familia

For the Patient

You should always carry . . .

1 your diabetic ID card.
2 candies.

Para el Paciente

Debe llevar *siempre* . . .

1 su tarjeta de diabético (a).
2 dulces.

For Family Members

Help the patient . . .

1 follow his (her) diet.
2 remember to take his (her) insulin.

Para los Parientes

Ayude al paciente a que . . .

1 *siga* su dieta.
2 *recuerde* usar su insulina.

INSUFFICIENT INSULIN— FOR THE PATIENT

INSUFICIENTE INSULINA—PARA EL PACIENTE

If . . .

1 you *do not use enough* insulin,
2 if you do not follow your diet, you may . . .

1 be thirsty.
2 have dry skin.
3 feel nauseated.
4 vomit.
5 faint.
6 have a headache.
7 breathe deeply or rapidly.

Si . . .

1 *no se pone suficiente* insulina,
2 *no come* lo indicado, puede tener . . .

1 *mucha* sed.
2 piel seca.
3 náusea.
4 vómitos.
5 desmayos.
6 dolor de cabeza.
7 respiraciones *profundas* o *rápidas*.

8 urinate frequently.

If THIS happens, you must . . .
1 ask someone for help.
2 call your doctor.
3 have someone take you to the hospital.
4 call 911.

INSUFFICIENT INSULIN— FOR FAMILY MEMBERS

If you notice ____[2]
1 assist the patient with his (her) instructions.
2 call the doctor.
3 take the patient to the hospital.
4 call 911.

INSULIN EXCESS— FOR THE PATIENT

If . . .
1 you use too much insulin,
2 you do not follow your diet,
3 you let too much time pass without eating after taking your insulin,

8 necesidad de *orinar con más frecuencia.*

Si ESTO le sucede debe . . .
1 pedir ayuda a alguien.
2 llamar a su médico.
3 pedir que le lleven al hospital.
4 llamar al nueve uno uno.

INSUFICIENTE INSULINA— PARA LOS PARIENTES

Si nota ____[2]
1 ayude al paciente con con sus instrucciones.
2 llame al médico.
3 lleve al paciente al hospital.
4 llame al nueve uno uno.

EXCESO DE INSULINA—PARA EL PACIENTE

Si . . .
1 se pone demasiado insulina,
2 no come lo indicado,
3 deja pasar mucho tiempo sin comer después de ponerse la insulina,

[2]Repeat the symptoms listed under Insufficient Insulin—for the Patient on page 97.

4 you exercise too much,
5 you work too much,

you may . . .

1 feel hungry.
2 be weak.
3 have cold sweats.
4 have blurred vision.
5 be nervous.
6 be dizzy.
7 feel confused.
8 have a headache.
9 faint.
10 have palpitations.

If THIS happens, you must . . .

1 eat or drink something sweet immediately.
2 ask someone for help.
3 call your doctor.
4 have someone take you to the hospital.
5 call 911.

INSULIN EXCESS— FOR FAMILY MEMBERS

If you notice _____[3]

1 assist the patient with his instructions.
2 call the doctor.
3 take the patient to the hospital.
4 call 911.

4 hace ejercicio excesivo,
5 trabaja demasiado,

puede tener . . .

1 hambre.
2 debilidad.
3 sudor frío.
4 visión nublada.
5 nerviosismo.
6 mareos.
7 confusión.
8 dolor de cabeza.
9 desmayos.
10 palpitaciones.

Si ESTO le sucede, debe . . .

1 comer o beber algo dulce inmediatamente.
2 pedir ayuda de alguien.
3 llamar a su médico.
4 pedir que le lleve al hospital.
5 llame al nueve uno uno.

EXCESO DE INSULINA— PARA LOS PARIENTES

Si nota _____[3]

1 ayude al paciente con sus instrucciones.
2 llame a su médico.
3 lleve al paciente al hospital.
4 llame al nueve uno uno.

[3]Repeat the symptoms listed under Insulin Excess—for the Patient on page 99.

If the patient is . . .

1 convulsing
2 unconscious

NEVER give him (her)
anything to eat or drink.

Si el paciente está . . .

1 convulsionando (a)
2 inconsciente

NUNCA le de nada de
comer o beber.

8.2 INDEX OF THERA-PEUTIC GROUPS

I am going to treat you with
a medicine for your illness.

I am going to treat you
with . . .

analgesic that is . . .

1 habit-forming.
2 not habit-forming.

anesthetic that is . . .

1 local.
2 general.

antacid
antialcohol agent

antiallergen[4]

INDICE DE GRUPOS TERAPÉUTICOS

Voy a tratarle con una
medicina para mejorar su
enfermedad.

Le voy a tratar con . . .

una medicina *para el dolor
que* . . . (a medicine for
pain that . . .)

1 puede *producir* hábito.
2 no *produce* hábito.

un anestésico . . .

1 local.
2 general.

un antiácido
una medicina que le ayudará
a *dejar de tomar alcohol* (a
medicine that will help you
stop drinking alcohol)
una medicina *para las
alergias*[4]

---

[4]If no English translation is given in parentheses, then the Spanish phrase is just an explanation of what the drug does:
antiallergen . . . medicine against allergies.
antidiarrheal . . . medicine against diarrhea.

antiamebic agent	una medicina *para las amebas*
antianginal agent	una medicina *para el dolor del pecho* (a medicine for chest pain)
antiarrhythmic agent	una medicina *para mejorar el ritmo de su corazón* (a medicine that improves the rhythm of your heart)
antiarthritic agent	una medicina *para el reumatismo*
antibiotic	antibiótico
anticancer agent	una medicina *para el cáncer*
anticoagulant	una medicina que *evita la formación de coágulos*
anticonvulsant	una medicina *para las convulsiones*
antidepressant	una medicina *para la depresión*
antidiarrheal	una medicina *para la diarrea*
antiemetic	una medicina *para los vómitos* (a medicine for vomiting)
antifungal agent	una medicina *para la infección* por *hongos*
antigout agent	una medicina *para la gota*
antihelminthic	una medicina *para las lombrices* (a medicine for worms)
antihemorrhagic agent	una medicina que *evita la hemorragia*
antihistamine	un *antihistamínico*
antihyperlipemic agent	una medicina *para bajar . . .* (a medicine that lowers . . .) 1 el colesterol (cholesterol) 2 los triglicéridos (triglycerides)

antihypertensive agent	una medicina *para bajar su presión* (a medicine that lowers blood pressure)
anti-inflammatory agent	una medicina *para la inflamación*
antimalarial agent	una medicina *para la malaria*
antimanic agent	una medicina *para equilibrar* su estado *emocional* (a medicine to balance your emotional state)
anti–motion-sickness agent	una medicina *para . . .* (a medicine for . . .) 1 mareo (dizziness) 2 vértigo (vertigo)
antinauseant	una medicina *para la náusea*
antiparkinson agent	una medicina *para su temblor* (a medicine for your tremor)
antipsychotic agent	una medicina *para modificar su estado mental* (a medicine to modify your mental state)
antipyretic agent	una medicina *para bajar la fiebre* (a medicine that lowers fever)
antiseptic	antiséptico
antispasmodic	una medicina *para aliviar los espasmos*
antithyroid agent	una medicina *para bajar la función de la tiroide* (a medicine that lowers thyroid function)
antituberculous agent	una medicina *para tuberculosis*
antitussive agent . . .	una medicina *para la tos* . . . (a cough medicine . . .)

1 with codeine	1 *con codeína*
2 without codeine	2 *sin codeína*
antiviral agent	*una medicina paro las infecciones virales*
appetite depressant	*una medicina para quitar el apetito*
appetite stimulant	*una medicina para estimular el apetito*
bronchodilator	*una medicina para respirar más fácilmente* (a medicine that helps you breathe more easily)
decongestant	*un descongestionante*
digestant	*una medicina para mejorar la digestión* (a medicine that improves digestion)
digitalis	*una medicina para mejorar la función del corazón* (a medicine that improves the function of your heart)
diuretic	*una medicina para orinar más* (a medicine that makes you urinate more)
emetic	*una medicina para vomitar* (a medicine that makes you vomit)
fertility agent	*una medicina que le ayudará a tener hijos* (a medicine that helps you have children)
hematinic	*una medicina para las anemias* (a medicine that improves anemias)
hematopoietic	*una medicina para producir más sangre* (a medicine that produces more blood)
insulin that is . . .	*insulina de acción . . .*
1 short-acting	1 *corta*
2 medium-acting	2 *mediana*
3 long-acting	3 *larga*

laxative	un laxante
muscle relaxant	una medicina que *relaja los músculos*
oral contraceptive	un *anticonceptivo oral*
oral hypoglycemic	una medicina *para la diabetes* (a medicine for diabetes)
oxytocic	una medicina que *aumenta las contracciones del útero* (a medicine that increases uterine contractions)
sedative	un sedante
steroids	esteroides . . .
1 androgens	1 *hormonas masculinas* (male hormones)
2 corticosteroid that is . . .	2 corticoesteroides . . .
a topical	a tópicos
b oral	b orales
c injectable	c inyectables
3 estrogens	3 *hormonas femeninas* (female hormones)
thyroid drug	una medicina *para aumentar la función del tiroides* (a medicine that increases thyroid function)
tranquilizer	un tranquilizante
vaccine for ____ [5]	una *vacuna* para ____ [5]
vasodilator that is . . .	una medicina *para mejorar la circulación* . . . (a medicine that improves circulation of . . .)
1 general	1 del cuerpo (the body)
2 coronary	2 del corazón
3 cerebral	3 del cerebro
vitamins	vitaminas

---

[5]Fill in the blank with the appropriate vaccine.

Chapter 9
CONTRACEPTION
AND PATIENT
INSTRUCTION

This chapter contains nine sections. Each one is devoted to instructions for the use of a specific method of contraception. This topic is complicated in any language, and unfortunately, the instructions in Spanish are also long. Whenever possible, the instructions are simplified into a series of phrases. Many of the instructions have been left open ended so that the health worker may substitute his or her preferred instruction.

Example:	*Ejemplo:*
Don't douche for ____ hours after intercourse.[1]	No emplee duchas vaginales hasta después de ____ horas des sus relaciones.[1]
Do you presently use contraception?	Usa anticonceptivos actualmente?
Do you use . . .	Usa . . .

1 the contraceptive pill . . .	1 la píldora anticonceptiva . . .
a minipill (progestin only)?	a la píldora mini (solamente progesterona)?
b 28-day combination pill (progestin and estrogen)?	b la píldor combinada de 28 días (progesterona y estrógeno)?
c 3-month combination pill (estrogen and progestin)?	c la píldora combinada de 3 meses (progesterona y estrógeno)?
2 the contraceptive ring?	2 el anillo anticonceptivo?
3 the contraceptive patch?	3 el parche anticonceptivo?
4 the Depo-Provera shot?	4 la inyección de Depo-Provera?
5 the diaphragm?	5 el diafragma?
6 the IUD?	6 el dispositivo intrauterino?
7 vaginal foam?	7 espuma vaginal?
8 vaginal suppository?	8 supositorios vaginales?
9 condoms?	9 condones?
10 the rhythm method?	10 el método del ritmo?

[1]Throughout this chapter, fill in the blank with your own specific instructions.

11 the method of withdrawal?	11 el método de retirarse antes de eyacular?
12 abstinence?	12 abstinencia?
13 the morning-after pill?	13 la píldora de la mañana siguiente?

Have you had . . .	Le han efectuado . . .
1 a tubal ligation?	1 una ligadura de trompas?
2 a vasectomy?	2 una vasectomía?

Would you like to have . . .	Le gustaría tener . . .
1 a tubal ligation?	1 una ligadura de trompas?
2 a vasectomy?	2 una vasectomía?

Are you satisfied with your present method of contraception?	Está satisfecha (o) con su método actual?

9.1 INSTRUCTIONS FOR THE BIRTH CONTROL PILL

INSTRUCCIONES PARA LA PÍLDORA ANTICONCEPTIVA

It is important to follow all the instructions when taking the pill.	Es importante seguir todas las instrucciones cuando usa la píldora.
Take the pill at the same time each day.	Tome la píldora a la misma hora cada día.

It can be in the . . .	Puede ser por la . . .
1 morning.	1 mañana.
2 evening.	2 noche.

If you forget to take a pill, take it as soon as you remember it.	Si se le olvida tomar una píldora, debe tomarla enseguida que se acuerde.
Then take the next pill at the usual hour.	Luego, tome la otra píldora a la hora acostumbrada.

With the pill you may . . .	Con la píldora quizá . . .
1 retain water.	1 retendrá agua.

2 have . . .
   a enlarged breasts.
   b tender breasts.
3 get headaches.
4 become irritable.
5 have increased libido.

6 have decreased libido.

7 develop discoloration of
   the skin of your face.

8 need a change in your
   contact lens prescription.

9 you may have breakthrough
   bleeding the first month
   or two.

If you develop any of the
following problems, stop the
pill immediately and call your
doctor . . .

1 chest pain of any kind.

2 shortness of breath.
3 sudden severe headache.

4 vomiting.
5 dizziness.
6 disturbances of vision
   or speech.
7 pain, redness or swelling
   of an arm or leg.

8 severe abdominal pain.
9 yellow discoloration of skin
   or eyes.
10 severe depression.

2 tendrá senos . . .
   a más grandes.
   b dolorosos.
3 tendrá dolor de cabeza.
4 estará más irritable.
5 aumentarán sus deseos
   sexuales.
6 disminuirán sus deseos
   sexuales.
7 experimentará una
   decoloración de la piel
   de la cara.
8 necesita cambiar la
   receta de sus lentes de
   contacto.
9 podrá tener espacios
   mientras sangra el
   primer o segundo mes.

Si se le presenta alguno de
estos problemas, deje de
tomar la píldora
inmediatamente y llame a su
doctor . . .

1 dolor del pecho de
   cualquier tipo.
2 falta de aire.
3 dolor de cabeza severo
   o repentino.
4 vómitos.
5 mareos.
6 problemas para ver o
   hablar.
7 dolor, enrojecimiento o
   hinchazón de un brazo
   o una pierna.
8 dolor de estómago severo.
9 decoloración amarilla
   de la piel o los ojos.
10 depresión severa.

There are three types of pills. You have the . . .	Hay tres clases de píldoras. Usted tiene . . .
1 "mini" pill (progestin only).	1 la píldora "mini" (solamente progesterona).
2 28-day combination pill (estrogen and progestin).	2 la píldora combinada de 28 días (estrógeno y progesterona).
3 3-month combination pill (estrogen and progestin)	3 la píldora combinada de 3 meses (estrógeno y progesterona).

9.1.1 Mini Pill

La Píldora Mini

1 Take the first pill on the first day of your period.	1 Tome la primera píldora el primer día de su regla.
2 Day 1 of your period is the first day you bleed.	2 El primer día de su regla es el primer día que sangra.
3 Take the pills daily.	3 Tome las píldoras diariamente.
4 Begin the next package on the next day after you finish the other pack.	4 Empiece el próximo paquete el próximo día después de terminar el otro paquete.
5 If your period does not start, begin the next pack as indicated even if your period has not started.	5 Si su regla no viene, continúe con el próximo paquete como está señalado aunque no comience su regla.

9.1.2 28-Day Combination Pill

La Píldora Combinada de 28 Días

1 Day 1 of your period is the first day you bleed.	1 El primer día de su regla es el primer día que sangra.

2 Take the first pill . . .

a the fifth day of your period
OR
b the first Sunday after your
period begins

OR
c the first day of your period.
3 Take THESE daily for
3 weeks.

4 Take THESE daily for the
next 7 days then begin a
new pack.

5 Your period will begin on
the second or third day
after you begin the last row
of pills (THESE taken for
7 days).

6 You must take a pill every
day.
7 If your period does not start,
begin the next pack as
indicated.

2 Tome la primera píldora
en . . .

a el quinto día de su regla
O
b el primer domingo
después del comienzo
de su regla
O
c el primer día de su regla.
3 Tome ÉSTAS
diariamente durante tres
semanas.

4 Tome ÉSTAS
diariamente durante los
próximos siete días
luego comience un
paquete nuevo.

5 Su regla vendrá el
segundo o tercer día
después de empezar la
última fila de píldoras
(ÉSTAS tomadas por
siete días).

6 Hay que tomar una
píldora cada día.
7 Si su regla no viene,
continúe con el
próximo paquete como
está señalado.

9.1.3 3-Month Combination Pill

1 Take the first pill on . . .
a the fifth day of your period

OR
b the first Sunday after your
period begins

La Píldora Combinada de 3 Meses

1 Tome la píldora en . . .
a el quinto día de su
regla

O
b el primer domingo
después del comienzo
de su regla

OR

c the first day of your period.

2 Take a pill every day.

3 There are 2 colors of pills in each pack . . .

a 84 of THIS COLOR.

b 7 of THIS COLOR.

4 You should have your period during the last 7 days when you are taking THESE pills.

5 You will only have 4 periods per year.

6 You may have breakthrough bleeding during the first 2 or 3 months.

O

c el primer día de su regla.

2 Tome una píldora cada día.

3 Hay dos colores de píldoras en cada paquete . . .

a ochenta y cuatro de ESTE COLOR.

b siete de ESTE COLOR.

4 Su regla vendrá durante los últimos siete días cuando esté tomando ESTAS píldoras.

5 Solamente tendrá cuatro reglas por año.

6 Podrá tener espacios mientras sangra durante los primeros dos o tres meses.

9.2 INSTRUCTIONS FOR THE CONTRACEPTIVE RING

INSTRUCCIONES PARA EL ANILLO ANTICONCEPTIVO

1 The contraceptive ring works like the birth control pill.

2 Place the ring inside the vagina . . .
a the first day of your period

OR

b the first Sunday after your period begins.

3 Remove the ring at the end of 3 weeks.

1 El anillo anticonceptivo funciona como la píldora anticonceptiva.

2 Meta el anillo dentro de la vagina . . .
a en el primer día de su regla

O

b el primer domingo después de que comience su regla.

3 Quítese el anillo después de tres semanas.

4 Leave the ring out for
1 week.
5 You will have your period
the week the ring is not
used.
6 After the 1-week break,
insert the next ring.
7 Do the same each month
with a new ring.
8 Store extra rings in the
refrigerator.

4 No use el anillo durante
una semana.
5 Su regla vendrá durante
la semana que no usa
el anillo.
6 Después de la semana
libre del anillo, meta el
próximo anillo.
7 Cada mes haga lo
mismo con un anillo
nuevo.
8 Guarde los otros anillos
en el refrigerador.

9.3 INSTRUCTIONS FOR THE CONTRACEPTIVE PATCH

INSTRUCCIONES PARA EL PARCHE ANTICONCEPTIVO

1 The contraceptive patch
works like the birth
control pill.
2 Apply the patch to the skin
of either the . . .
a abdomen.
b buttocks.
c outer arms.

d upper torso.

3 Apply the patch . . .
a once per week.
b always the same day of
the week.
c 3 weeks in a row.

4 During the fourth week do
not use the patch.

1 El parche anticonceptivo
funciona como la
píldora anticonceptiva.
2 Aplique el parche a la
piel ya sea . . .
a del abdomen.
b de los glúteos.
c de la parte de atrás de
los brazos.
d de la parte de arriba
del cuerpo.

3 Aplique el parche . . .
a una vez por semana.
b siempre el mismo día
de la semana.
c tres semanas
consecutivas.

4 Durante la cuarta
semana no use el
parche.

5 You will have your period during the fourth week.	5 Su regla vendrá durante la cuarta semana.
6 Repeat the same each month will a new patch.	6 Cada mes haga lo mismo con un parche nuevo.

9.4 INSTRUCTIONS FOR THE DEPO-PROVERA SHOT

INSTRUCCIONES PARA LA INYECCIÓN DE DEPO-PROVERA

1 Depo-Provera, or "the shot," is an intramuscular shot of progesterone that keeps you from ovulating. It is one of the most effective reversible contraceptives available to women.

1 Depo-Provera, o "la inyección," es una inyección intramuscular de progesterona que previene la ovulación. Es uno de los modos más efectivos de contracepción reversible para las mujeres.

2 We will give you an injection in your . . .
a arm.
b buttock.

2 Le pondremos una inyección en sus . . .
a brazos.
b glúteos.

3 You will receive an injection every 11 to 13 weeks.

3 Recibirá una inyección cada once o trece semanas.

4 You can have irregular bleeding or spotting. This will decrease over time. After the first year you may stop having any periods at all.

4 Puede tener períodos irregulares o manchar. Esto disminuirá con el tiempo. Después del primer año, podrá dejar de tener su período del todo.

5 With Depo-Provera you may . . .
a gain weight.
b have headaches.
c experience depression.

5 Con Depo-Provera puede . . .
a ganar peso.
b tener dolor de cabeza.
c tener depresiones.

d have a temporary decrease in bone density.

6 Most women are able to get pregnant within a year after their last Depo-Provera injection.

7 Like oral contraceptives, Depo-Provera does not protect against sexually transmitted diseases.

d tener una disminución temporal en la densidad de sus huesos.

6 La mayoría de las mujeres pueden quedar embarazadas después de un año de haber recibido su última inyección de Depo-Provera.

7 Como las píldoras anticonceptivas, Depo-Provera tampoco la protege contra las enfermedades transmitidas sexualmente.

9.5 INSTRUCTIONS FOR THE DIAPHRAGM

You can put it in place ____ hours before having intercourse.
Don't forget to put the special cream on and in the diaphragm before putting it in.

You can remove the diaphragm ____ hours after intercourse.

INSTRUCCIONES PARA EL DIAFRAGMA

Puede ponérselo ____ hora(s) antes de tener relaciones sexuales.
No se olvide de poner la crema especial sobre y en el diafragma antes de ponérselo.
Puede quitarlo ____ horas después de las relaciones.

9.6 INSTRUCTIONS FOR THE IUD

Would you like to use an IUD?

I can fit one for you.

INSTRUCCIONES PARA EL DISPOSITIVO INTRUTERINO

Le gustaría usar el dispositivo intrauterino?
Puedo colocarle uno.

When the IUD is in its proper place, the string will always be the same length. You can check the length by inserting your finger. Try IT now. Your IUD needs to be changed in _____ years.

Cuando está bien colocado el hilo siempre tendrá el mismo largo. Puede comprobarlo introduciendo el dedo. HágaLO ahora. Hay que cambiar su dispositivo intrauterino dentro de _____ años.

9.7 INSTRUCTIONS FOR THE CONDOM, FOAM, AND VAGINAL SUPPOSITORY

INSTRUCCIONES PARA EL PRESERVATIVO, LA ESPUMA, Y EL SUPOSITORIO VAGINAL

9.7.1 The Condom

El Condón

1 When used alone, the condom is not 100% effective to prevent pregnancy. It is best to use a condom plus vaginal foam or a vaginal suppository.

1 Cuando se usa solo, el preservativo (el condón) no es cien por ciento seguro para evitar el embarazo. Es mejor usar el condón junto con la espuma vaginal o un supositorio vaginal.

2 The condom is the only method, other than abstinence, to prevent venereal infection.

2 El preservativo es la única manera de evitar las infecciones venéreas, a no ser que se abstenga completamente de tener relaciones.

3 Always use a condom for . . .
a oral sex.
b vaginal sex.
c anal sex.

3 Siempre use un condón para . . .
a sexo oral.
b sexo vaginal.
c sexo anal.

4 Do not use a condom more than once.

4 No use un condón más de una vez.

5 Always use a condom made of latex, unless you or your partner are allergic.

6 Do not use condoms made of . . .
a lambskin.
b natural membranes.

7 Read the package label to be sure the condom is latex.

8 As soon as the penis is erect, put the condom on.

9 Leave space at the top of the condom to collect semen.

5 Siempre use un condón hecho de látex, a menos que usted o su pareja sean alérgicos.

6 No use condones hechos de . . .
a piel de cordero.
b membranas naturales.

7 Lea el paquete para asegurarse que es hecho de látex.

8 En seguida que el pene se ponga erecto, colóquese el condón.

9 Deje un espacio en la punta del condón para recoger el semen.

9.7.2 Vaginal Foam and Suppositories

1 When used alone . . .
a vaginal foam is not very effective to prevent pregnancy.

b vaginal suppositories are not very effective to prevent pregnancy.

2 They are better than using nothing at all.

3 It is best to use a condom plus vaginal foam or a vaginal suppository.

4 Insert the . . .
a foam _____ hour(s) before intercourse.

Espuma Vaginal y Supositorios

1 Cuando se usa sola . . .
a la espuma vaginal no es muy segura para evitar el embarazo.

b los supositorios vaginales no son muy seguros para evitar el embarazo.

2 Es mejor usarlos que no usar nada.

3 Es mejor usar un condón junto con la espuma vaginal o un supositorio vaginal.

4 Póngase . . .
a la espuma _____ hora(s) antes del acto sexual.

b vaginal suppository ____
hour(s) before
intercourse.

5 The man should wear the
condom whenever he
enters the vagina, not only
during intercourse.

6 Don't douche for ____
hours after intercourse. It
inactivates the effect of the
foam and suppository.

b el supositorio vaginal
____ hora(s) antes
del acto sexual.

5 El hombre debe usar el
condón cada vez
que el pene tiene
contacto con la vagina,
no sólo durante el
verdadero acto sexual.

6 No emplee duchas
vaginales hasta después
de ____ horas de sus
relaciones. Inactiva los
efectos de la espuma y
del supositorio vaginal.

9.7 INSTRUCTIONS FOR THE RHYTHM METHOD

This method is only advisable
for a woman who has very
regular periods.

Counting the first day of your
menses as day one, do not
have intercourse from day
____ to day ____.
If you have intercourse during
days ____ to ____, you
should use another type of
barrier contraception.

INSTRUCCIONES PARA EL MÉTODO DEL RITMO

Este método es aconsejable
sólo para las mujeres que
tienen su regla
puntualmente.
Contando el primer día de
su regla como día uno, no
tenga relaciones sexuales del
día ____ hasta el día ____.
Si tiene relaciones sexuales
durante los días ____ a
____, tiene que utilizar otro
método de barrera de
contracepción.

9.9 INSTRUCTIONS FOR THE MORNING-AFTER PILL

1 Would you like to have a
prescription for the
morning-after pill?

INSTRUCCIONES PARA LA PILDORA DEL DÍA SIGUIENTE

1 Desea una receta para la
píldora del día siguiente?

2 Here is a prescription to have just in case you have unprotected sex (or a condom breaks).

3 Take the first pill as soon as possible.

4 Take the second pill 12 hours after.

2 Aquí tiene una receta, por si acaso tiene relaciones sexuales sin protección (o se rompe un condón).

3 Tome la primera píldora enseguida que puede.

4 Tome la segunda píldora doce horas después.

Chapter 10
PREGNANCY AND DELIVERY

The four sections of this chapter cover history of past pregnancies and deliveries, present pregnancy and delivery, and instructions for breast-feeding.

10.1 HISTORY OF PAST PREGNANCIES AND DELIVERIES

HISTORIA DE PARTOS Y EMBARAZOS ANTERIORES

How many times have you been pregnant?

Cuántas veces ha estado embarazada?

How many children do you have?

Cuántos hijos tiene?

Did you breast-feed them?

Les dio el pecho?

Have you ever had . . .

Ha tenido . . .

1 babies that were . . .
   a large?
   b small?
   c premature?

1 niños . . .
   a grandes?
   b pequeños?
   c prematuros?

d congenitally
malformed?
2 multiple births . . .

a twins?
b more than two?
3 a forceps delivery?
4 a cesarean?
5 a child that was born . . .

a feet first?
b with the cord around
the neck?
6 a child that was born
dead?
7 a child that died shortly
after birth?

8 problems with the
placenta?
9 a postpartum hemorrhage?

10 a miscarriage?
11 an abortion?
12 with your pregnancy have
you ever had . . .

a diabetes?
b high blood pressure?

c leg swelling?

d liver problems?

How many weeks pregnant
were you when you had . . .

1 the abortion?
2 the miscarriage?

d con defectos de
nacimiento?
2 nacimientos
múltiples . . .
a gemelos (as)?
b más de dos?
3 un parto con fórceps?
4 una cesárea?
5 un niño que haya
nacido . . .
a de pies?
b con el cordón
alrededor del cuello?
6 un niño que haya
nacido muerto?
7 un niño que haya
muerto poco después
de nacer?
8 algún problema con la
placenta?
9 una hemorragia
después del parto?
10 un aborto espontáneo?
11 un aborto provocado?
12 con el embarazo ha
tenido problemas
con . . .
a diabetes?
b alta presión de
sangre?
c hinchazón de las
piernas?
d el hígado?

Cuántas semanas de
embarazo tenía cuando tuvo
el . . .

1 el aborto provocado?
2 el aborto espontáneo?

3 the problem?	3 el problema?
How long was your labor with the . . .	Cuánto le duró el trabajo de parto con . . .
1 first child?	1 su primer niño?
2 other children?	2 sus otros niños?
How much did your children weigh?	Cuánto pesaron sus niños?

10.2 PRESENT PREGNANCY

EMBARAZO ACTUAL

I am going to examine you.	La voy a *examinar*.
What is the date of your last period?	Cuándo fue su última regla?
Do you have OR have you had . . .	Tiene O ha tenido . . .
1 anxiety?	1 ansiedad?
2 depression?	2 depresion?
3 irritability?	3 irritabilidad?
4 sleepiness?	4 sueño?
5 insomnia?	5 insomnio?
6 headaches?	6 *dolores* de cabeza?
7 vision problems?	7 molestias de la vista?
8 convulsions?	8 convulsiones?
9 nausea?	9 náusea?
10 vomiting?	10 vómitos?
11 constipation?	11 estreñimiento?
12 loss of appetite?	12 *pérdida* de apetito?
13 craving for special food?	13 antojos?
14 urinary problems?	14 molestias urinarias?
15 a lot of vaginal secretions?	15 mucho flujo vaginal?
16 vaginal spotting?	16 sangre por la vagina?
17 tiredness?	17 cansancio?
18 low back pain?	18 dolor de espalda?
19 swelling of your feet?	19 *hinchazón* de los pies?
20 varicose veins?	20 *várices*?

21 hemorrhoids?	21 hemorroides?
22 difficulty in breathing?	22 *dificultad* para respirar?
23 high blood pressure?	23 *presión* alta?
You are ____ weeks pregnant.	Usted tiene ____ semanas de embarazo.
You need to have . . .	Necesita tener . . .
1 an ultrasound.	1 un ultrasonido.
2 routine blood tests.	2 pruebas rutinarias de sangre.
3 a stress test.	3 una prueba para chequear el niño.
4 an amniocentesis.	4 un amniocentesis.
Was this a planned pregnancy?	Estaba planeando este embarazo?
Do you want to . . .	Quiere . . .
1 continue with the pregnancy?	1 seguir con el embarazo?
2 have an abortion?	2 tener un aborto provocado?
Do you want to breast-feed this child?	Quiere darle de mamar a este niño?
Do you have any hereditary diseases in your family?	Tiene alguna enfermedad hereditaria en su familia?
Are you taking . . .	Está tomando . . .
1 any medications?	1 alguna medicina?
2 vitamins?	2 vitaminas?
What are they?	Cuáles son?

10.3 PRESENT DELIVERY

PARTO ACTUAL

How close together are the pains?	Cada cuánto le vienen los dolores?

How long do they last?	Cuánto le duran?
Do you know if . . .	Sabe si . . .
1 a lot of water has come out?	1 ha salido mucho agua?
2 blood has come out?	2 ha salido sangre?
I am going to examine you.	La voy a examinar.
You are ____ centimeters dilated.	Tiene ____ centímetros de cuello.
Do you need to urinate?	Tiene deseos de orinar?
I am going to . . .	Voy a . . .
1 shave you.	1 rasurarle.
2 clean you.	2 limpiarle.
3 give you an enema.	3 darle un enema.
Do you want something for the pain?	Desea alguna medicina para el dolor?
Would you like epidural anesthesia?	Desea anestesia epidural?
This will monitor . . .	Esto va a chequear . . .
1 the baby's heart rate.	1 el pulso del niño.
2 your contractions.	2 sus contracciones.
You will have to . . .	Tendrá que . . .
1 wait patiently.	1 esperar tranquilamente.
2 tell me when you have a pain.	2 avisarme cuando tenga dolor.
3 slide closer to the edge of the table.	3 acercarse al borde de la mesa.
4 put your legs up HERE.	4 poner las piernas AQUÍ.
5 relax your muscles.	5 relajar sus músculos.
6 calm yourself.	6 calmarse.
7 breathe slowly through your mouth.	7 respirar lentamente por la boca.
8 pant.	8 jadear.
9 push only when you are told.	9 empujar solo cuando le diga.

10	conserve your strength.	10	conservar su fuerza.
11	rest between pains.	11	descansar cuando no tenga dolor.
12	turn on your side.	12	descansar en su lado.
13	have an episiotomy.	13	tener una episiotomía.
14	have stitches.	14	tener puntos.

The baby is having a problem.
You need an emergency cesarean section.
Breath this oxygen.
You will need general anesthesia.

El niño tiene unos problemas.
Necesita una cesárea urgente.
Respire este oxígeno.
Necesita anestesia general.

It is a . . .

Es . . .

1 boy.
2 girl.

1 un niño.
2 una niña.

He (she) weighs _____ pounds and _____ ounces.

Pesa _____ libras y _____ onzas.

He (she) is healthy.

Es sano (a).

Would you like to see your baby?

Le gustaría ver a su niño (a)?

10.4 INSTRUCTIONS FOR BREAST-FEEDING

INSTRUCCIONES PARA AMAMANTAR

To keep your milk flowing . . .

Para mantener la producción de su leche . . .

1 rest adequately.

1 descanse adecuadamente.

2 eat a balanced diet.

2 coma una dieta balanceada.

3 drink plenty of fluids including milk.

3 tome bastante líquidos, incluyendo leche.

Before you breast-feed . . .	Antes de amamantar . . .
1 wash your hands.	1 lávese las manos.
2 wash your breasts and nipples.	2 lávese los pechos y los pezones.
You can breast-feed . . .	Puede amamantar . . .
1 sitting in a chair.	1 sentada en una silla.
2 lying down.	2 acostada.
Place the child in your arms . . . [1]	Ponga al niño en sus brazos . . . [1]
1 so that the baby's head is higher than its stomach.	1 para que la cabeza del niño esté más alta que el estómago.
2 so that the baby is well supported.	2 para que el niño esté seguro.
3 so that the whole baby (not just the head) is turned toward you.	3 para que todo el cuerpo del niño (no sólo la cabeza) esté doblado hacia usted.
4 touch your nipple to the baby's mouth and insert the nipple when the baby's mouth opens.	4 toque el labio del niño con su pezón y ponga el pezón dentro de la boca del niño cuando la abra.
To better position yourself you may want to . . .	Para ponerse en una mejor posición, se puede . . .
1 place balnkets under the baby's head to have the baby at the level of the breast.	1 poner cobijas debajo de la cabeza del niño para tenerlo al mismo nivel de su pecho.
2 place your feet on a stool to raise your knees and bring the baby closer to your breast.	2 poner sus pies en un banquillo para levantar sus rodillas y acercar al niño a su pecho.

[1]See figure 10.1 page 126.

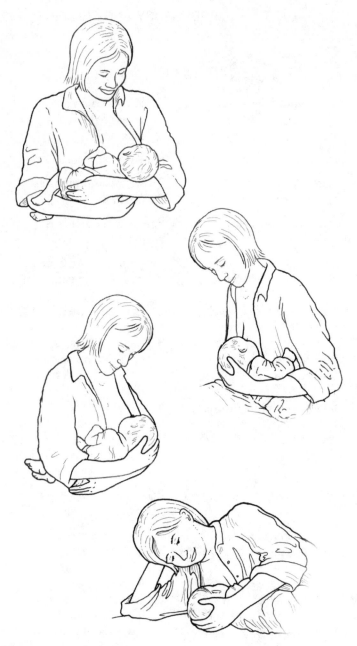

Figure 10.1

Breast-feed . . .

1 when the baby is hungry.

2 every 1, 2, or 3 hours.

3 for about 10 to 20 minutes each time.

Breast-feed until the breast is empty then change to the other breast.

If one breast is enough, use the other breast the next time.

Call your doctor if . . .

1 you have any problems.

2 you feel the baby is not eating well.

3 the baby develops a rash or colic.

Amamante . . .

1 cuando el niño tenga hambre.

2 cada una, dos o tres horas.

3 entre diez a veinte minutos cada vez.

Amamante al niño de un pecho hasta que se vacíe, luego cámbielo al otro pecho.

Si un pecho es suficiente, use el otro la próxima vez.

Llame a su médico si . . .

1 tiene algún problema.

2 siente que el niño no está comiendo suficiente.

3 el niño tiene erupción o cólico.

Chapter 11
PHYSICAL AND SEXUAL ABUSE AND RAPE

11.1 PHYSICAL AND SEXUAL ABUSE

In your relationship with your spouse or friend, does her (she) . . .

1   shout frequently?
2   threaten you physically or verbally?
3   try to control your behavior?
4   have abusive or harmful sex with you?
5   threaten your children?
6   interfere with your ability to visit or speak with other family members or friends?

ABUSO FISICO Y SEXUAL

En su relación con su esposo (a) o amigo (a), él (ella) . . .

1   grita frecuentemente?
2   lo (a) amenaza fisicamente o verbalmente?
3   trata de controlar su comportamiento?
4   tiene relaciones sexuales abusivas o peligrosas?
5   amenaza a sus niños?
6   interfiere con su habilidad de visitar o hablar con sus familiares o amigos?

7 place limitations on your other activities?	7 impone límites sobre sus otras actividades?
Were these bruises caused by . . .	Fueron estos moretones causados por . . .
1 falling?	1 una caída?
2 bumping into something?	2 golpeándose con algo?
3 someone hurting you?	3 alguien haciéndole daño?
4 someone trying to rape you?	4 alguien tratando de violarla (o)?
Do you know who hurt you . . .	Sabe quién le hizo daño . . .
1 spouse?	1 esposo (a)?
2 friend?	2 amigo (a)?
3 stranger?	3 extraño?
4 other?	4 otro?
Did they have a weapon?	La persona estaba armada?
When did this happen?	Cuándo le pasó?
What time?	A qué hora?
Where did this happen?	Dónde le pasó?
Has this happened before?	Le ha pasado esto antes?
Did you call the police?	Llamó a la policía?
Would you like me to call them now?	Le gustaría que la llame ahora?
Are you safe?	Está segura(o)?
Do you have a safety plan?	Tiene un plan de seguridad?
Do you have someone to call?	Tiene a alguien que pueda llamar?

11.2 RAPE / VIOLACIÓN SEXUAL

My nurse will be with us while we talk.	Mi enfermera estará aquí mientras hablamos.
Do you know who raped you . . .	Sabe quién la(o) violó . . .

1 spouse?
2 friend?
3 stranger?
4 other?

Do you know his name?
Please, write it HERE

_____.

When did this happen?
What time?
Where did this happen?
Are these the clothes you
were wearing when you
were raped?

Have you showered or bathed
since the attack?

Did your attacker have a
weapon?

Please show me where you
were touched or hurt.

Did you scratch your attacker?

Have you had any alcohol or
used any drugs?

When?
What?

During the rape was there . . .

1 vaginal penetration?
2 anal penetration?
3 oral penetration?

Was the penetration with . . .
1 the penis?
2 a foreign object?

1 esposo(a)?
2 amigo(a)?
3 extraño(a)?
4 otro?

Sabe su nombre?
Por favor, escríbalo AQUÍ

_____.

Cuándo le pasó?
A qué hora?
Dónde le pasó?
Esta es la misma ropa que
usted tenía cuando sufrió
la violación?

Se ha bañado o duchado
desde la violación?

La persona que la(o) violó
tenía alguna arma?

Por favor, enséñeme dónde
la(o) tocaron o le hicieron
daño.

Rasguñó al que la(o) atacó?

Ha tomado alcohol o
drogas?

Cuándo?
De qué tipo?

Durante la violación
hubo . . .

1 penetración vaginal?
2 penetración anal?
3 penetración oral (por la
   boca)?

La penetración fue con . . .
1 el pene?
2 un objeto extraño?

If it was penetration with the penis, did he . . .	Si fue penetración con el pene, sabe si . . .
1 wear a condom?	1 usó un condón?
2 ejaculate?	2 eyaculó?
Do you have any bruises or cuts?	Tiene algunos morados o cortadas?
Please, show me where.	Por favor, enséñeme dónde.
My nurse will be here while . . .	Mi enfermera estará aquí mientras . . .
1 we talk.	1 hablamos.
2 I examine you.	2 yo la (o) examino.
When was your last period? Is there any chance that you are pregnant? I am going to examine you. I will examine for . . .	Cuándo fue su última regla? Hay alguna posibilidad de que esté embarazada? La (o) voy a examinar. La (o) examino por . . .
1 bruises.	1 morados.
2 cuts.	2 cortadas.
I will take pictures of any bruises or cuts. I need to take samples from beneath your fingernails.	Voy a sacar fotos de los morados y las cortadas. Necesito tomar muestras debajo de sus uñas.
I need a urine sample.	Necesito una muestra de orina.
I need to do a pelvic exam.	Tengo que hacer un examen pélvico.
I need to . . .	Necesito . . .
1 trim samples of pubic hair.	1 cortar muestras del pelo pubico.
2 insert the speculum into your vagina.	2 poner el especulo dentro de la vagina.
3 take samples of semen.	3 tomar muestras de semen.

4 culture for infection such as . . .
a Gonorrhea.
b Chlamydia.

4 hacer cultivo para . . .
a Gonorrea.
b Chlamydia.

Were you forced to perform oral sex?

La forzaron a hacer sexo oral?

I need to take a sample from your mouth and throat.
I need to do a blood test for AIDS and syphilis.

Necesito tomar una muestra de la boca y de la garganta.
Necesito hacer una prueba de sangre para el SIDA y para sífilis.

I am going to give you some medicine to prevent infection.
Do you want a pregnancy prevention pill?

Voy a darle una medicina para prevenir infección.
Desea una píldora para evitar el embarazo?

Would you like me to call a . . .

Desea que llame a . . .

1 friend?
2 relative?
3 Rape Crisis Center?

1 un amigo(a)?
2 un pariente?
3 la oficina del Centro de Crisis de Violación?

You are safe now.
It is not your fault you were raped.

Está a salvo ahora.
No es su culpa que la violaron.

Chapter 12
POISONING
AND PATIENT
INSTRUCTION

This chapter is designed to aid the health worker in cases of intoxication. It contains a list of the more common poisonous agents, immediate instructions for the patient or other party to follow, and a list of general symptoms associated with the various intoxicants.

The text is written in two styles. The first is a set of instructions directed to a third party. For example, a parent calls or brings the child to the hospital because she suspects he (she) has swallowed a poison. The second style is the same set of instructions directed to the patient him- or herself.

The chapter ends with general instructions designed to explain how to help avoid future problems of this nature.

12.1 COMMON INTOXICANTS

INTOXICANTES COMUNES

What did he (she, you)
swallow?
[I don't know.]¹
[I think it is . . .

Qué tomó?

[No sé.]¹
[Creo que es . . .

1 a medicine . . .
    a aspirin.
    b amphetamines.
    c barbiturates.
    d tranquilizers.
    e antiallergen.
    f cough syrup.
    g contraceptives.
    h antiseptics.
	1 una medicina . . .
	    a aspirina.
	    b anfetaminas.
	    c barbitúricos.
	    d tranquilizantes.
	    e antialérgenicos.
	    f jarabe para la tos.
	    g anticonceptivos.
	    h antisépticos.

2 alcohol.	2 alcohol.

3 a cleaning agent . . .
    a Clorox.
    b furniture polish.
	3 un líquido limpiador . . .
	    a cloro.
	    b una cera para
	      muebles.

    c a disinfectant.   c un desinfectante.
    d a detergent.   d un detergente.
4   an insecticide.   4   un insecticida.
5   a hair dye.   5   un tinte para el pelo.
6   lead from . . .   6   plomo de . . .
    a paint.   a pintura.
    b metal toys.   b juguetes de metal.
    c batteries.   c baterías.
7   a plant.   7   una planta.
8   a mushroom.   8   un hongo.
9   spoiled food . . .   9   una comida pasada . . .
    a milk and milk   a leche y derivados.
      products.
    b canned goods.]   b productos enlatados.]

When did he (she, you)
swallow it?

Cuándo lo tragó?

---

¹The square brackets indicate possible responses by the patient or third party.

How much did he (she, you) swallow?

Call THIS number _____.

Cuánto tragó?

Llame a ESTE número _____.

12.2 INSTRUCTIONS DIRECTED TO A THIRD PARTY

INSTRUCCIONES DIRIGIDAS A OTRA PERSONA

Do the following . . .

1 give him (her) . . .
  a milk.
  b egg whites.
  c vinegar.
  d strong tea.
  e black coffee.
  f mineral oil.
  g antacid.
2 induce vomiting with . . .
  a your finger.
  b mustard and water.
  c salt and water.
3 bring him (her) to the hospital immediately.
4 call 911.

Haga lo siguiente . . .

1 déle . . .
  a leche.
  b clara de huevos.
  c vinagre.
  d té fuerte.
  e café negro.
  f aceite mineral.
  g antiácido.
2 hágale vomitar con . . .
  a su dedo.
  b agua con mostaza.
  c agua con sal.
3 llévelo al hospital inmediatamente.
4 llame al nueve uno uno.

12.3 INSTRUCTIONS DIRECTED TO THE PATIENT

INSTRUCCIONES DIRIGIDAS AL PACIENTE

Do the following . . .

1 drink . . .
  a milk.
  b egg whites.
  c vinegar.
  d strong tea.
  e black coffee.
  f mineral oil.
  g antacid.

Haga lo siguiente . . .

1 tome . . .
  a leche.
  b clara de huevos.
  c vinagre.
  d té fuerte.
  e café negro.
  f aceite mineral.
  g antiácido.

2	induce vomiting with . . .	2	hágale vomitar con . . .
a	your finger.	a	su dedo.
b	mustard and water.	b	agua con mostaza.
c	salt and water.	c	agua con sal.
3	come to the hospital immediately.	3	venga al hospital inmediatamente.
4	call 911.	4	llame al nueve uno uno.

12.4 COMMON SYMPTOMS

SÍNTOMAS COMMUNES

Does he (DO you) have OR has he (have you) had . . .

Tiene O Ha tenido . . .

1	dizziness?	1	mareo?
2	irritability?	2	irritabilidad?
3	sleepiness?	3	mucho sueño?
4	insomnia?	4	insomnia?
5	depression?	5	depresión?
6	excitability?	6	excitación?
7	convulsions?	7	convulsiones?
8	paralysis?	8	parálisis?
9	confusion?	9	confusión mental?
10	incoordination?	10	pérdida de coordinación?
11	constipation?	11	estreñimiento?
12	nausea?	12	náusea?
13	vomiting?	13	vómitos?
14	diarrhea?	14	diarrea?
15	abdominal pain?	15	cólicos abdominales?
16	headache?	16	dolor de cabeza?
17	respiratory difficulty?	17	dificultad respiratoria?
18	palpitations?	18	palpitaciones?
19	blue fingers?	19	dedos morados?
20	blue lips?	20	labios morados?
21	small pupils?	21	pupilas pequeñas?
22	large pupils?	22	pupilas grandes?
23	blurred vision?	23	vista nublada?
24	a dry mouth?	24	sequedad de la boca?

12.5 INSTRUCTIONS FOR PREVENTION OF FUTURE INTOXICATIONS

ALWAYS keep all medicines and poisons . . .

1 away from children.
2 in a locked cabinet.
3 in a high place.
4 in their original containers.
5 labeled clearly.

NEVER keep medicines and poisons . . .

1 with food.
2 in food containers such as . . .
   a milk bottles.
   b pop bottles.

INSTRUCCIONES PARA LA PREVENCIÓN DE INTOXICACIONES FUTURAS

SIEMPRE guarde medicinas y substancias peligrosas . . .

1 donde los niños no las alcancen.
2 en un gabinete cerrado con llave.
3 en un sitio alto.
4 en su caja original.

5 con una etiqueta clara.

NUNCA guarde medicinas y substancias peligrosas . . .

1 donde hay comida.
2 en un recipiente para la comida como . . .
   a botellas de leche.
   b botellas de soda.

Chapter 13
AIDS AND PATIENT INSTRUCTIONS

13.1 INFORMATION FOR THE PATIENT

AIDS is an infection caused by a virus.
The virus is called HIV.

HIV is transmitted by blood products and sexual relations.
HIV weakens the body's defenses to infections.

It can take years of infection with HIV before one develops AIDS.

INFORMACIÓN PARA EL PACIENTE

SIDA es una infección causada por un virus.
El virus se llama VIH o virus de SIDA.
VIH se transmite por productos de sangre y relaciones sexuales.
VIH debilita las defensas del cuerpo contra las infecciones.
Puede estar infectado con VIH por años antes de tener SIDA.

13.2 RISK FACTORS FOR HIV

Have you . . .

1 had sexual relations with many different people?
2 had sexual relations with a person infected with HIV?
3 had oral sex?
4 had anal sex?
5 been raped?
6 been sexually abused?
7 shared needles with a person who uses drugs?

8 received a blood transfusion before 1985?

9 been artificially inseminated before 1985?

10 ever had a sexually transmitted disease?

When was your last sexual contact?
Do you know the person you had sex with?

FACTORES DE RIESGO DEL VIH

Ha tenido . . .

1 relaciones sexuales con varias personas?
2 relaciones sexuales con alguien infectado con el virus del SIDA?
3 sexo oral?
4 sexo por el ano?
5 una violación sexual?
6 abuso sexual?
7 experiencias compartiendo agujas con alguien que usa drogas?

8 una transfusión de sangre antes del año mil novecientos ochenta y cinco?

9 inseminación artificial antes del año mil novecientos noventa y cinco?

10 una enfermedad que fue transmitida sexualmente?

Cuándo fue su último contacto sexual?
Conoce a la persona con quien tuvo sexo?

13.3 EVALUATION FOR HIV

There is a blood test to detect whether you have been infected by the AIDS virus.

EVALUACÍON PARA VIH

Hay un examen de sangre para detectar si usted está infectado por el virus que causa SIDA.

I will . . .

1 call you with the results.

2 see you HERE about the results.

The blood test is not perfect, but it is extremely accurate.

I need your permission to perform this blood test.

The results of the blood test will be kept confidential.

Sometimes it is necessary to repeat the test in a few months.

Would you like to speak to someone who speaks your own language about HIV and AIDS?

I will give you their telephone number.

I will set up an appointment for you.

I will have the results of your blood test in _____ days.

Yo . . .

1 lo llamaré con los resultados.

2 lo veré AQUÍ con los resultados.

El examen de sangre no es perfecto, pero es muy exacto.

Necesito su permiso para hacer este examen de sangre.

El resultado del examen de sangre será confidencial.

De vez en cuando es necesario repetir el examen de sangre después de unos meses.

Desea hablar con alguien sobre VIH y SIDA en su propio idioma?

Le voy a dar su numero de teléfono.

Voy a hacer una cita para usted.

Tendré los resultados de su examen de sangre dentro de _____ días.

13.4 DISEASES ASSOCIATED WITH AIDS

Although there is no cure for AIDS at this time, there are many helpful treatments.

ENFERMEDADES ASOCIADAS CON EL SIDA

Aunque en este momento no hay cura para el SIDA, hay muchos tratamientos efectivos.

Patients with AIDS sometimes get infected with viruses, bacteria, or funguses. PCP, or pneumocystis, is a type of lung infection that many AIDS patients get.

There is inhaled and intravenous medicine for PCP. Kaposi's sarcoma is a tumor that some AIDS patients get.

The lesions of Kaposi's sarcoma can affect the skin, intestines, lungs, or brain.

There are medical treatments, including chemotherapy, for Kaposi's sarcoma.

Pacientes con SIDA algunas veces sufren de infecciones de virus, bacteria, u hongos. PCP, o pneumocystis, es una infección del pulmón de la cual sufren muchos pacientes con SIDA. Hay medicina inhalada e intravenosa para PCP.

El sarcoma de Kaposi es un tumor del cual sufren algunos pacientes con SIDA. Las lesiones del sarcoma de Kaposi se encuentran en la piel, en los intestinos, en los pulmones, o en el cerebro. Hay tratamientos médicos, incluyendo la quimioterapia contra el sarcoma de Kaposi.

13.5 HIV PREVENTION

You must be careful not to infect your mate with the HIV virus.

You must use a condom when having intercourse. Condoms are helpful to prevent sexually transmitted diseases, including HIV, but are not 100 percent effective.

PREVENCIÓN DEL VIH

Tiene que tener cuidado para no infectar a su compañero(a) con el virus del SIDA. Tiene que usar un condón cuando tiene coito. El condón ayuda a prevenir la transmisión de enfermedades venéreas, incluyendo el VIH, pero no es cien por ciento efectivo.

The only prevention for AIDS is sexual abstinence.

Friends and family members with whom you are not intimate are not at risk of getting AIDS from you.

If you use intravenous drugs, you must not share needles with anyone.

A woman infected with HIV can transmit the virus to her baby . . .

1 during pregnancy.
2 during delivery.
3 with breast-feeding.

La única manera de prevenir el SIDA es abstenerse sexualmente.

Amigos y miembros de la familia con los cuales usted no tiene relaciones intimas no tienen peligro de contraer el SIDA de usted.

Si usa drogas intravenosas, nunca comparta agujas con nadie.

Una mujer infectada por el virus del SIDA puede transmitirlo a su bebé . . .

1 durante el embarazo.
2 durante el parto.
3 si le da pecho al bebé.

13.6 INSTRUCTIONS FOR CONDOM USE

INSTRUCCIONES PARA EL USO DEL CONDÓN

Always use a condom for . . .

1 oral sex.
2 vaginal sex.
3 anal sex.

Do not use a condom more than once.

Always use a condom made of latex unless you or your partner are allergic.

DO not use condoms made of . . .

1 lambskin.
2 natural membranes.

Siempre use un condón para . . .

1 sexo oral.
2 sexo vaginal.
3 sexo por el ano.

No use un condón más de una vez.

Siempre use un condón hecho de látex a menos que usted o su pareja sean alérgicos.

No use condones hechos de . . .

1 piel de cordero.
2 membranas naturales.

Read the package label to be sure the condom is latex.	Lea el paquete para asegurarse que el condón está hecho de látex.
As soon as the penis is erect, put the condom on.	En seguida que el pene se ponga erecto colóquese el condón.
Leave space at the top of the condom to collect semen.	Deje un espacio en la punta del condón para recoger el semen.

Chapter 14
GERIATRIC
EVALUATION[1]

Chapter 14 is devoted to the specialty of geriatric medicine. The chapter allows you to evaluate the specific functional problems encountered by the geriatric patient. A mini mental status examination is also provided.

14.1 SOCIAL BACKGROUND

DATOS SOCIALES

How old are you?

Cuántos años tiene usted?

Do you live . . .

Vive . . .

1 alone?

1 solo (a)?

[1]Prepared in consultation with Dr. Rafael J. Leo for the third edition of Medical Spanish.

2 with family . . .	2 con familia . . .
a husband (wife)?	a esposo (a)?
b brother (sister)?	b hermano (a)?
c grandson (granddaughter)?	c nieto (a)?
d nephew (niece)?	d sobrino (a)?
e cousin?	e primo (a)?
f son-in-law (daughter-in-law)?	f yerno (a)?
3 with a friend?	3 con un amigo (a)?

How long have you lived . . .	Cuánto tiempo ha vivido . . .
1 alone?	1 solo (a)?
2 with family?	2 con familia?
3 with a friend?	3 con un amigo (a)?

Are you . . .	Es . . .
1 single?	1 soltero (a)?
2 married?	2 casado(a)?
3 widowed?	3 viudo (a)?
4 divorced?	4 divorciado (a)?
5 separated?	5 separado (a)?

For how long . . .	Por cuánto tiempo . . .
1 weeks?	1 semanas?
2 months?	2 meses?
3 years?	3 años?

Do you have family (friends) nearby?	Tiene familia (amigos) cerca?
Who is it?	Quién es?
Where do they live?	Dónde viven ellos?

Do you speak (visit) with them . . .	Habla (visita) con ellos . . .
1 daily?	1 cada día?
2 weekly?	2 cada semana?
3 monthly?	3 cada mes?
4 annually?	4 cada año?

5 only on holiday?	5 solamente días de fiesta?
Whom do you call in case of emergency?	A quién llama en caso de emergencia?
What is their telephone number?	Cuál es su número de teléfono?
Do you know the number for emergency?	Sabe el número a llamar en caso de emergencia?
Can you hear the telephone ring?	Puede oír el teléfono cuando suena?
Do you have electricity in your home?	Tiene electricidad en su casa?
Do you have a car?	Tiene un carro?
Have you had any accidents recently?	Ha tenido un accidente recientemente?
Can you use . . .	Puede utilizar . . .
1 the bus?	1 el bus?
2 the train?	2 el tren?
3 taxicabs?	3 un taxi?

14.2   SOCIAL HABITS

14.2.1   *Alcohol Use*

HÁBITOS SOCIALES

Uso de Alcohol

Do you drink alcohol . . .	Bebe alcohol . . .
1 daily?	1 cada día?
2 weekly?	2 cada semana?
How much each day . . .	Cuánto bebe al día . . .
1 glass?	1 vaso?
2 bottle?	2 botella?
3 cup?	3 copa?
Do you drink when you are . . .	Bebe cuando está . . .
1 alone?	1 solo (a)?

2 sad?	2 triste?
3 depressed?	3 deprimido (a)?
4 happy?	4 alegre?
5 in a social situation only?	5 en una reunión social solamente?
Do you think you have a drinking problem?	Cree que tiene problemas de alcoholismo?
Would you like help?[2]	Quiere ayuda?[2]

14.2.2 Smoking Habits	**Hábitos de Tabaco**
Do you smoke OR have you ever smoked . . .	Fuma O ha fumado . . .
1 cigarettes?	1 cigarrillos?
2 pipe?	2 pipa?
3 cigars?	3 cigarros?
4 marijuana?	4 marihuana?
How much do you smoke a day?	Cuánto fuma al día?
How long have you been smoking?	Hace cuánto tiempo que fuma?
Have you ever tried to stop?	Ha tratado de dejar de fumar?
Would you like to stop?	Le gustaría dejar de hacerlo?

14.2.3 Sleeping Habits	**Hábitos Para Dormir**
Do you ever have problems sleeping?	Tiene problemas para dormir?
What time do you get up in the morning?	A qué hora se levanta por la mañana?

[2]See page 170 for further questions about alcohol use.

Is your sleep . . .	Duerme . . .
1 restful?	1 tranquilo (a)?
2 interrupted?	2 inquieto (a)?
How many hours do you sleep each night?	Cuántas horas duerme cada noche?
Do you take naps during the day?	Toma siestas durante el día?
How many?	Cuántas?
How long?	Cuánto tiempo?
Do you take pills or alcohol to sleep?	Toma píldoras o alcohol para dormir?
How long have you done this?	Hace cuánto tiempo que lo hace?

14.3 MEDICAL BACKGROUND

DATOS MÉDICOS

How many medications do you take daily?	Cuántas medicinas toma cada día?
Do you have your medicines here with you?	Tiene sus medicinas aquí ahora?
Please show them to me.	Por favor, déjeme verlas.
Have you had vaccination for . . .	Se ha vacunado contra . . .
1 tetanus?	1 el tétano?
2 pneumococcal pneumonia	2 neumonía de neumococo?
3 influenza?	3 influenza?
Have you had . . .	Ha tenido . . .
1 a mammogram?	1 una mamografía?
2 sigmoidoscopy?	2 una sigmoidoscopía?
3 colonoscopy?	3 una colonoscopía?

4 a gynecologic examination?	4 un examen ginecológico?
5 a prostate exam?	5 un examen de la próstata?
Was the last one within . . .	El ultimo fue hace . . .
1 six months?	1 seis meses?
2 a year?	2 un año?
3 three years?	3 tres años?
4 five years?	4 cinco años?
Where was it done?	Dónde lo tuvo?
What medical problems do you have?	Qué enfermedades tiene?
1 high blood pressure?	1 presión alta?
2 hyperlipidemia . . .	2 hiperlipidemia . . .
a high cholesterol?	a colesterol elevado?
b high triglycerides?	b triglicéridos elevados?
3 heart disease?	3 enfermedad del corazon?
4 heart attack?	4 ataque de corazón?
5 stroke?	5 derrame cerebral?
6 varicose veins?	6 várices?
7 thrombophlebitis?	7 tromboflebitis?
8 arteriosclerosis?	8 arterioesclerosis?
9 arthritis?	9 artritis?
10 kidney disease?	10 enfermedad de los riñones?
11 diabetes?	11 diabetes?
12 cancer? What type?	12 cáncer? Qué tipo?
13 bronchitis?	13 bronquitis?
14 tuberculosis?	14 tuberculosis?
15 asthma?	15 asma?
16 pneumonia?	16 neumonía?
17 bleeding tendencies?	17 tendencias a sangrar?
18 anemias . . .	18 anemias . . .
a sickle cell?	a células falciformes?
b thalassemia?	b talasemia?
c iron deficiency?	c deficiencia de hierro?

19	convulsions?		19	convulsiones?
20	mental retardation?		20	retraso mental?
21	psychiatric problems?[3]		21	problemas psiquiátricos?[3]
22	emotional problems?		22	problemas emocionales?
23	glaucoma?		23	glaucoma?
24	cataracts?		24	cataratas?
25	congenital defects?		25	defectos de nacimiento?

Do you have pain?

Tiene dolor?

Where is the pain?

Donde está el dolor?

How long have you had it?

Hace cuánto tiempo que lo tiene?

Did it develop . . .

Se inició . . .

1 slowly?
2 suddenly?

1 lentamente?
2 de repente?

Is this (Was that) the first time that you have (had) this type of pain?

Es (Era) la primera vez que le aparece (aparecía)?

When was the first time?

Cuándo fue la primera vez?

How long does (did) the pain last each time?

Cuánto le dura (duraba) cuando le viene (venía)?

Is (Was) it . . .

Es (Era) un dolor . . .

1 severe pain?
2 mild?
3 moderate?
4 sharp?
5 intermittent?
6 constant?
7 boring?
8 colicky?

1 severo?
2 leve?
3 moderado?
4 agudo?
5 intermitente?
6 constante?
7 penetrante?
8 cólico?

[3]See Chapter 15 for a detailed psychiatric interview.

9 shooting?	9 fulgurante?
10 burning?	10 quemante?
11 cramping?	11 como un calambre?
12 pressurelike?	12 opresivo?
Where is (was) the pain?	Dónde le duele (dolía)?
Show me with one finger.	Señáleme con un dedo.
Has (Did) the pain changed (change) location?	Ha cambiado (Cambió) de lugar?
Where did the pain begin?	Dónde le empezó?
Where does (did) it hurt . . .	Dónde le duele (dolía) . . .
1 the most?	1 más?
2 the least?	2 menos?
Does (Did) the pain radiate?	Se corre (corría) el dolor?
From where to where?	Hacia dónde?
Do (Did) you have the pain . . .	Tiene (Tenía) el dolor . . .
1 all the time?	1 todo el tiempo?
2 in the morning?	2 por la mañana?
3 in the afternoon?	3 por la tarde?
4 at night?	4 por la noche?
5 before eating?	5 antes de comer?
6 after eating?	6 después de comer?
7 while eating?	7 mientras come (comía)?
8 when it is (was) cold?	8 cuando hace (hacía) frío?
9 when it is (was) hot?	9 cuando hace (hacía) calor?
10 when it is (was) humid?	10 cuando está (estaba) húmedo?
11 when you are (were) . . .	11 cuando está (estaba) . . .
a upset?	a molesto (a)?
b worried?	b preocupado (a)?
12 when you exercise (exercised)?	12 cuando hace (hacía) ejercicio?

13 when you urinate
    (urinated) . . .
    a at the beginning?
    b the whole time?

    c at the end?
14 when you defecate
    (defecated)?
15 when you have (had)
    sexual relations?
16 when you swallow
    (swallowed) . . .
    a liquids?
    b solids?
    c both?
17 when you . . .
    a stand (stood)?
    b sit (sat) down?

    c lie (lay) down?

    d walk (walked)?
    e climb (climbed) stairs?

    f bend (bent) over?

Is (Was) there anything that
makes (made) the pain . . .

1 better?
2 worse?

What is (was) it?

Is (Was) there anything else
that accompanies (accompanied)
the pain?

Does (Did) the pain go away
when you rest (rested)?

13 cuando orina
    (orinaba) . . .
    a al empezar?
    b durante todo el
      tiempo que orina?
    c al terminar?
14 cuando evacúa
    (evacuaba)?
15 cuando tiene (tenía)
    relaciones sexuales?
16 cuando traga
    (tragaba) . . .
    a líquidos?
    b sólidos?
    c ambos?
17 cuando . . .
    a está (estaba) de pie?
    b está (estaba) sentado
      (a)?
    c está (estaba) acostado
      (a)?
    d camina (caminaba)?
    e sube (subía)
      escaleras?
    f se agacha
      (agachaba)?

Hay (Había) algo que . . .

1 lo alivie (aliviara)?
2 lo aumente (aumentara)?

Qué es (era)?

Hay (Había) otras molestias
que acompañan
(acompañaban) el dolor?

Se alivia (aliviaba) el
dolor al descansar?

Do (Did) you awake at night from this pain?	Lo despierta (despertaba)?
Do (Did) you take anything for the pain?	Toma (Tomaba) algo para el dolor?
Does (Did) it help?	Lo alivia (aliviaba)?
Does (Did) it make it worse?	Lo aumenta (aumentaba)?
For the pain do you take . . .	Para el dolor toma . . .

1 aspirin? 1 aspirina?
2 nonsteroidal anti-inflammatory drugs? 2 antiinflamatorio no esteroide?
3 narcotic pain medication? 3 narcóticos?

How is your appetite?	Comó está su apetito?
Has your weight . . .	Su peso . . .

1 increased? 1 ha subido?
2 decreased? 2 ha bajado?
3 stayed the same? 3 es igual?

Do you have problems with . . .   Tiene problemas . . .

1 vision? 1 con los ojos?
2 hearing? 2 con los oídos?
3 walking? 3 para caminar?
4 balance? 4 de equilibrio?
5 bowel incontinence? 5 para retener la orina?
6 bladder incontinence? 6 para retener el excremento?

Do you have an interest in sexual activity?	Tiene interés en actividades sexuales?
Do you have sexual intercourse?	Tiene relaciones sexuales?
Do you have OR have you had any problems with . . .	Tiene O ha tenido problemas con . . .

1 erection? . . . 1 la erección? . . .
   a There is (was) none?   a No la tiene (tenía)?
   b Is (Was) it difficult to achieve?   b Le cuesta (costaba)?

c Is (Was) it painful?

2 ejaculation? . . .
   a There is (was) none?
   b Is (Was) it difficult to achieve?
   c Is (Was) it premature?
   d Is (Was) it painful?
   e Is (Was) it bloody?
3 orgasm? . . .
   a There is (was) none?
   b Is (Was) it difficult to achieve?
   c Is (Was) it painful?
4 the quantity of genital secretions? . . .
   a Is (Was) it excessive?
   b Is (Was) it too little?

Are you OR have you been . . .

1 physically abused?
2 sexually abused?

c Es (Era) dolorosa?

2 la eyaculación? . . .
   a No hay (había)?
   b Le cuesta (costaba)?
   c Es (Era) prematura?
   d Es (Era) dolorosa?
   e Es (Era) con sangre?
3 el orgasmo? . . .
   a No tiene (tenía)?
   b Le cuesta (costaba)?

   c Es (Era) doloroso?
4 la cantidad de secreciones genitales?
   a Es (Era) excesiva?
   b Es (Era) poca?

Sufre O ha sufrido de . . .

1 abuso físico?
2 abuso sexual?

14.4 FUNCTIONAL ASSESSMENT

EVALUACIÓN FUNCIONAL

Do you have problems . . .

1 getting out of bed by yourself?
2 getting out of a chair by yourself?
3 getting out of a bath or shower by yourself?
4 going up and down stairs?

5 getting washed by yourself?
6 brushing your teeth?

7 getting dressed by yourself?

Tiene problemas . . .

1 para levantarse de la cama solo (a)?
2 para levantarse de una silla solo (a)?
3 para salir del baño o la ducha solo (a)?
4 para subir o bajar las escaleras solo (a)?
5 para lavarse solo (a)?
6 para cepillarse los dientes?
7 para vestirse solo (a)?

8	with household chores?	8	para hacer tareas de la casa?
9	shopping for yourself?	9	para ir de compras solo (a)?
10	falling down?	10	cayéndose?
11	with fatigue?	11	de cansancio?
12	concentrating?	12	para concentrarse?
13	understanding?	13	para entender?
14	getting lost?	14	perdiéndose?
15	remembering?	15	para recordar . . .
	a names?		a nombres?
	b dates?		b datos?
	c phone numbers?		c números de teléfono?
	d directions?		d direcciones?
	e the past?		e el pasado?
16	losing things?	16	perdiendo las cosas?
17	preparing your meals?	17	para preparar sus comidas?
18	eating your meals?	18	para comer solo (a)?

Do you have . . .   Tiene . . .

1	pain with chewing?	1	dolor al masticar?
2	your own teeth?	2	los dientes propios?
3	dentures?	3	dientes postizos?
4	problems with how your dentures fit?	4	problemas con los dientes postizos?
5	trouble with . . .	5	problemas con la comida . . .
	a solid food?		a sólida?
	b liquids?		b líquida?
6	diet changes because of these problems?	6	cambios en la dieta a causa de estos problemas?

Do you pay the . . .   Paga . . .

1	rent alone?	1	la renta solo (a)?
2	bills alone?	2	las cuentas solo (a)?

Does anyone help you?   Alguien le ayuda?

Who?   Quién es?

14.5 MENTAL AND EMOTIONAL ASSESSMENT

Do you often feel OR have you felt . . .

1 afraid?
2 angry?
3 anxious?
4 bored?
5 depressed?
6 guilty?
7 happy to be alive?
8 hopeless?
9 isolated?
10 lonely?
11 sad?
12 your life is empty?
13 worthless?

Do you prefer to . . .

1 stay at home?
2 go out?
3 visit with people?
4 try new things?
5 meet new people?

What is the . . .

1 season?
2 day?
3 month?
4 year?
5 state?
6 city?

Please repeat these three objects . . .

1 house.
2 car.
3 book.

EVALUACIÓN MENTAL EMOCIONAL

Se siente O se ha sentido . . .

1 asustado (a)?
2 enojado (a)?
3 ansioso (a)?
4 aburrido (a)?
5 deprimido (a)?
6 culpable?
7 feliz de vivir?
8 sin esperanza?
9 aislado (a)?
10 solo (a)?
11 triste?
12 que su vida está vacía?
13 sin valor?

Prefiere . . .

1 estar solo (a)?
2 salir?
3 visitar a otros?
4 tratar cosas nuevas?
5 conocer a nueva gente?

Cuál es . . .

1 la estación del año?
2 el día?
3 el mes?
4 el año?
5 el estado?
6 la ciudad?

Por favor repita estas tres cosas . . .

1 casa.
2 carro.
3 libro.

Please remember these 3 objects . . .	Por favor recuerde estas tres cosas . . .
1 house.	1 casa.
2 car.	2 carro.
3 book.	3 libro.
I will ask you to repeat them later.[4]	Más tarde se las voy a preguntar.[4]
Please tell me the three objects.	Por favor, dígame las tres cosas.
Please subtract 7 from 100 and keep going down by seven.	Por favor, reste cien menos siete y siga restando siete.
93	noventa y tres
86	ochenta y seis
79	setenta y nueve
72	setenta y dos
65	sesenta y cinco
Please spell the word WORLD backwards.	Por favor, deletree la palabra MUNDO al revés.
Please say the days of the week backwards, starting with Saturday.	Por favor, dígame los días de la semana al revés, comenzando con el sábado.
Saturday	sábado
Friday	viernes
Thursday	jueves
Wednesday	miércoles
Tuesday	martes
Monday	lunes
Sunday	domingo
What are THESE objects . . .	Qué son ESTAS cosas . . .
1 wristwatch?	1 reloj de pulsera?
2 pencil (pen)?	2 lápiz (pluma)?

[4]The questioner should wait approximately five minutes before asking the patient to recall three objects.

Please follow these instructions . . .

Por favor, sigua estas instrucciones . . .

1 take this paper in your right hand.

1 tome el papel en su mano derecha.

2 fold it in half.

2 doble el papel por el medio.

3 place it on the floor

3 póngalo en el suelo.

4 point to the . . .
   a ceiling.
   b floor.
   c chair.

4 señale . . .
   a el cielo.
   b el piso.
   c el asiento.

Please . . .

Hágame el favor de . . .

1 read THIS and do what it says. (See Figure 1)

1 leer ESTO y hacer lo que dice.

**HAGA EL FAVOR DE
CERRAR LOS OJOS
(CLOSE YOUR EYES)**

Figure 1

2 write a sentence.

2 escribir una frase.

3 copy the drawing. (see Figure 2)

3 copiar este dibujo.

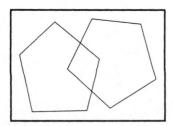

Figure 2

Please . . .

Por favor . . .

1 draw a large circle.

1 dibuje un círculo grande.

2 put numbers in the circle so that it resembles a clock.

2 ponga números en el circulo para que parezca un reloj.

3 have the clock hands show 11:10.	3 ponga las manos del reloj para que diga once y diez.

14.6 LETHALITY ASSESSMENT[5]	**EVALUACIÓN DEL INTENTO MORTAL**[5]

DO YOU HAVE THOUGHTS ABOUT HARMING YOURSELF?	**TIENE PENSAMIENTOS DE HACERSE DAÑO?**

DO YOU HAVE PLANS HOW YOU WOULD DO IT?	**TIENE IDEAS DE CÓMO LO HARÍA?**

DO YOU HAVE ACCESS TO WEAPONS?	**TIENE ACCESO A LAS ARMAS?**

HAVE YOU ATTEMPTED TO HARM YOURSELF BEFORE?	**HA TRATADO DE HACERSE DAÑO ANTES?**

Do you feel . . .

1 hopeless?
2 you would be better off dead?
3 others would be better off if you were dead?

4 you have problems controlling impulses?

Se siente . . .

1 sin esperanza?
2 qué sería mejor si estuviera muerto (a)?
3 qué sería mejor para los demás si usted estuviera muerto (a)?
4 que tiene problemas para controlar sus impulsos?

[5]Questions in bold are considered very important lines of inquiry and affirmative replies should prompt psychiatric referral.

DO YOU HAVE THOUGHTS ABOUT WANTING TO HARM SOMEONE ELSE?	**TIENE IDEAS DE HACERLE DAÑO A OTROS?**
DO YOU HAVE PLANS ON HOW YOU WOULD HARM THEM?	**TIENE IDEAS DE CÓMO LO HARÍA?**
DO YOU HAVE ACCESS TO THIS PERSON?	**PUEDE ENCONTRAR A ESA PERSONA?**
DO YOU HAVE ACCESS TO WEAPONS?	**TIENE ACCESO A LAS ARMAS?**
HAVE YOU HARMED SOMEONE PREVIOUSLY?	**LE HA HECHO DAÑO A OTRA PERSONA ANTES?**

Have you ever been charged with . . .

Le han acusado de . . .

1 assault?
2 homicide?

1 asalto?
2 homicidio?

Do you have trouble controlling unpleasant feelings, for example, anger, rage?

Tiene problemas para controlar las emociones malas, por ejemplo el enojo?

Chapter 15
THE PSYCHIATRIC
INTERVIEW[1]

This chapter provides questions for an in-depth psychiatric interview. Questions that are considered to be highly significant areas of inquiry are boldfaced and capitalized.

15.1 DEPRESSION	**DEPRESIÓN**
Has your mood been . . .	Su estado de animo ha sido . . .
1 sad?	1 triste?
2 irritable?	2 irritable?
3 tearful?	3 lagrimoso?

[1]Prepared in consultation with Dr. Rafael J. Leo for the third edition of Medical Spanish.

Have you felt this way for . . .	Se ha sentido así . . .
1 a few days?	1 pocos días?
2 a week?	2 una semana?
3 two to three weeks?	3 dos o tres semanas?
4 months?	4 meses?
5 as long as you can remember?	5 todo el tiempo que puede recordar?
Do you have interest in activities?	Tiene interés en actividades?
When something good happens do you feel happy?	Cuando algo bueno ocurre, se siente feliz?
Have you stopped many of your interests?	Ha dejado de hacer las cosas que le interesan?
Has there been a change in your interest in . . .	Ha cambiado su interés en . . .
1 watching TV?	1 mirar la televisión?
2 music?	2 la música?
3 reading?	3 leer?
4 shopping?	4 ir de compras?
5 socializing?	5 actividades sociales?
6 sex?	6 relaciones sexuales?
Has there been a change in your sleep?	Ha cambiado como duerme?
Is it . . .	Duerme . . .
1 increased?	1 más?
2 decreased?	2 menos?
Do you feel tired?	Se siente cansado (a)?
Do you have energy to complete day-to-day tasks?	Tiene energia para completar las tareas diarias?
Do you feel OR have you felt . . .	Se siente O ha sentido . . .
1 slowed down?	1 pesado (a)?
2 restless?	2 inquieto (a)?

Has there been a change in your . . .	Ha cambiado su . . .
1 appetite?	1 apetito?
2 weight?	2 peso?
Is it . . .	Ha . . .
1 increased?	1 subido?
2 decreased?	2 bajado?
Do you have difficulty . . .	Tiene dificultad para . . .
1 making decisions?	1 hacer decisiones?
2 concentrating on . . . a activities? b conversation?	2 concentrarse en . . . a las actividades? b la conversación?
Comparing yourself to others, do you have more problems with your memory?	Comparándose con los demás, tiene más problemas con la memoria?
Do you feel OR have you felt . . .	Siente O ha sentido . . .
1 guilty?	1 culpable?
2 badly about yourself?	2 vergüenza por si mismo?
3 hopeless about your future?	3 sin esperanza para el futuro?
4 worthless as you are?	4 que vale nada?
DO YOU THINK ABOUT DYING?[2]	**PIENSA EN LA MUERTE?**
DO YOU WISH YOU WERE DYING?	**DESEA MORIRSE AHORA?**
DO YOU WISH YOU WERE DEAD?	**DESEA ESTAR MUERTO (A) AHORA?**

[2]Questions in bold are considered very important lines of inquiry and affirmative replies should prompt psychiatric referral.

DO YOU THINK OF WAYS TO HARM YOURSELF?	**PIENSA EN CÓMO HACERSE DAÑO?**
Have you been treated by a doctor for this problem before?	Ha recibido tratamiento médico por este problema antes?
Have you been hospitalized for this problem before?	Ha estado hospitalizado por este problema antes?

15.2 MANIA — MANÍA

Do you feel OR have you felt . . .	Siente O ha sentido . . .
1 happier than usual?	1 más feliz que lo normal?
2 **IRRITABLE?**	2 **IRRITABLE?**
3 excited?	3 excitado (a)?
4 **ON-TOP-OF-THE-WORLD?**	4 **ENCIMA DEL MUNDO?**
5 there was nothing you couldn't do?	5 que puede hacer todo lo que quiere sin límites?
Do you have more energy than usual?	Tiene mas energía que lo normal?
Do you have less need for sleep lately?	Necesita dormir menos recientemente?

HAVE YOU FELT YOUR THOUGHTS WERE SO FAST YOU COULDN'T KEEP UP WITH THEM?	**HA SENTIDO QUE SUS PENSAMIENTOS VIENEN TAN RAPIDAMENTE QUE NO PUEDE CONTROLARLOS?**
Have others commented that they cannot follow your train of thought?	Le han dicho otros que no pueden entender sus ideas o sus pensamientos?
Have you been more talkative than usual?	Habla más de lo normal?

HAVE YOU BEEN TAKING ON MORE ACTIVITIES THAN USUAL?	ESTÁ HACIENDO MÁS ACTIVIDADES QUE LO NORMAL?

Are you . . .

1 working more?
2 more physically active?
3 spending more money?
4 spending money foolishly?
5 making excessive investments?
6 more sexually active?

Está . . .

1 trabajando más?
2 haciendo más actividad física?
3 gastando más dinero?
4 gastando dinero sin pensar?
5 haciendo inversiones excesivas?
6 participando más en actividades sexuales?

Have others commented that your behavior is excessive?

Le han dicho otros que su comportamiento es excesivo?

Have you felt this way for . . .

1 a few days?
2 a week?
3 two to three weeks?
4 months?
5 as long as you can remember?

Se ha sentido así . . .

1 pocos días?
2 una semana?
3 dos o tres semanas?
4 meses?
5 todo el tiempo que puede recordar?

Have you been treated by a doctor for this problem before?

Ha recibido tratamiento médico por este problema antes?

Have you been hospitalized for this problem before?

Ha estado hospitalizado (a) por este problema antes?

15.3 LETHALITY ASSESSMENT	EVALUACIÓN DEL INTENTO MORTAL
DO YOU HAVE THOUGHTS ABOUT HARMING YOURSELF?	**TIENE PENSAMIENTOS DE HACERSE DAÑO?**

DO YOU HAVE PLANS ON HOW YOU WOULD DO IT?	**TIENE IDEAS DE CÓMO LO HARÍA?**
DO YOU HAVE ACCESS TO WEAPONS?	**TIENE ACCESO A LAS ARMAS?**
HAVE YOU ATTEMPTED TO HARM YOURSELF BEFORE?	**HA TRATADO DE HACERSE DAÑO ANTES?**

Do you feel . . .

1 hopeless?
2 you would be better off dead?
3 others would be better off if you were dead?
4 you have problems controlling impulses?

Se siente . . .

1 sin esperanza?
2 que sería mejor si estuviera muerto (a)?
3 que sería mejor para los demás si usted estuviera muerto (a)?
4 que tiene problemas para controlar sus impulsos?

DO YOU HAVE THOUGHTS ABOUT WANTING TO HARM SOMEONE ELSE?	**TIENE IDEAS DE HACERLE DAÑO A OTROS?**
DO YOU HAVE PLANS ON HOW YOU WOULD HARM THEM?	**TIENE IDEA DE CÓMO LO HARÍA?**
DO YOU HAVE ACCESS TO THIS PERSON?	**PUEDE ENCONTRAR A ESTA PERSONA?**
DO YOU HAVE ACCESS TO WEAPONS?	**TIENE ACCESO A LAS ARMAS?**

HAVE YOU HARMED SOMEONE PREVIOUSLY?	**LE HA HECHO DAÑO A OTRA PERSONA ANTES?**
Have you ever been charged with . . .	Le han acusado de . . .
1 assault?	1 asalto?
2 homicide?	2 homicidio?
Do you have trouble controlling unpleasant feelings, for example, anger, rage?	Tiene problemas para controlar las emociones malas, por ejemplo el enojo?

15.4 PSYCHOSIS   PSICOSIS

15.4.1 Delusions

. . . of reference:

Do you feel as if, when the television or radio are on, they are sending messages intended just for you?	Se siente que la televisión o la radio, mandan mensajes solamente para usted?
Does it seem as if others, even those you don't know, are taking special notice of you?	Le parece que otros, incluyendo los extraños, le prestan atención especial?

. . . of grandeur:

Do you feel you have special powers or magical abilities no one else has?	Se siente que tiene habilidades especiales o mágicas que no tienen los demás?

. . . of persecution:

Do you feel others . . .	Se siente que otros . . .
1 are conspiring against you?	1 están conspirando contra usted?
2 are out to get you?	2 quieren castigarle?
3 may harm you?	3 quieren hacerle daño?

. . . of guilt:

Do you feel you have done something so bad that you feel you are being punished?	Se siente que ha hecho algo tan malo que le están castigando por hacerlo?
Do you feel responsible for events going on in the world . . .	Se siente responsable por acciones mundiales . . .
1 war?	1 las guerras?
2 starvation?	2 la inanición?

. . . of control:

Do you feel someone or something is controlling what you do from afar?	Se siente que alguien o algo está controlándole de lejos?

. . . of thought broadcasting:

Do you feel others can hear your thoughts without you saying or doing anything?	Se siente que otros pueden oír sus pensamientos aunque no diga o haga nada?
Do you feel people "read your mind" and know what you are thinking?	Se siente que otra gente puede "leer sus pensamientos" y entender lo que está pensando?

. . . of thought insertion:

Do you feel others can insert thoughts or ideas into your head?	Se siente que otros pueden poner ideas o pensamientos dentro de su cabeza?

. . . of depersonalization:

Does your body feel . . .	Siente su cuerpo . . .
1 strange?	1 extraño?
2 changed?	2 cambiado?
3 disconnected?	3 desconectado?

Do you feel as if you are in a movie, watching yourself go through the motions?

Se siente como si estuviera haciendo un papel en una película, mirándose a si mismo hacer las cosas?

. . . of unreality:

Does the world seem changed to you?

Le parece cambiado el mundo?

Is the appearance unchanged of . . .

Se ven igual que siempre . . .

1 people
2 cars
3 houses
4 trees
5 animals

1 la gente?
2 los carros?
3 las casas?
4 los árboles?
5 los animales?

appear as they usually do?

15.4.2 Hallucinations

Alucinaciones

DO YOU EVER SEE THINGS OTHERS WOULD BE UNABLE TO SEE?

VE USTED COSAS QUE OTROS NO PUEDEN VER?

DO YOU EXPERIENCE VISIONS?

TIENE VISIONES?

DO YOU HEAR VOICES OTHERS ARE UNABLE TO HEAR?

OYE USTED VOCES QUE OTROS NO PUEDEN OÍR?

DO YOU HEAR VOICES TALKING TO YOU OR ABOUT YOU?

OYE USTED VOCES QUE LE HABLAN O VOCES QUE HABLAN DE USTED?

DO YOU HEAR VOICES TELLING YOU/COMMANDING YOU TO DO THINGS?	**OYE USTED VOCES QUE LE MANDAN A HACER COSAS?**
Do you experience smells/odors other people don't notice?	Huele olores que nadie más huele?
Do you experience unusual sensations on your skin?	Siente sensaciones diferentes en la piel?
Do you experience crawling/creeping sensations on your skin?	Siente que algo se arrastra por su piel?
Do you experience unusual tastes in your mouth?	Prueba sabores diferentes en la boca?
Have you felt this way for a long time?	Hace tiempo que se siente así?
Have you been treated by a doctor for this problem before?	Ha recibido tratamiento médico por este problema antes?
Have you been hospitalized for this problem before?	Ha estado hospitalizado por este problema antes?

15.5 ALCOHOL AND DRUG USE	**USO DE ALCOHOL Y DROGAS**
Do you drink alcohol?	Toma alcohol?
Do you have periods when you get drunk?	Se emborracha?
Do you notice if it takes more for you to get drunk than it had previously?	Nota si tiene que beber más que antes para emborracharse?
When you stop drinking, do you have . . .	Cuando deja de tomar alcohol tiene . . .
1 tremors?	1 temblores?
2 sweating?	2 sudores?

3 nervousness?
4 difficulty sleeping?
5 nausea?
6 vomiting?

Do you drink . . .

1 to stop any of these
   symptoms?
2 for longer than you
   intended?
3 more than you intended?

Do you spend more time . . .

1 trying to acquire alcohol?
2 drinking?
3 hiding your drinking?

4 recovering from drinking
   episodes?

Because of your drinking
have you . . .

1 missed work?
2 been fired from work?
3 been suspended from
   school?
4 argued with your wife/
   husband?
5 been separated or
   divorced?
6 spent less time with
   your family?
7 been arrested?

Have you thought about . . .

1 stopping your drinking?
2 controlling your drinking?

3 nerviosismo?
4 dificultad para dormir?
5 nausea?
6 vómitos?

Toma alcohol . . .

1 para parar estos
   síntomas?
2 durante más tiempo del
   que había planeado?
3 en cantidades más
   grandes de las que había
   planeado?

Pasa más tiempo . . .

1 buscando alcohol?
2 tomando alcohol?
3 escondiendo su hábito
   de alcohol?
4 recuperándose de una
   borrachera?

Por culpa del alcohol . . .

1 ha faltado al trabajo?
2 ha perdido el trabajo?
3 le han suspendido de la
   escuela?
4 ha peleado con su
   esposa(o)?
5 se ha separado o
   divorciado?
6 ha pasado menos
   tiempo con la familia?
7 lo han arrestado?

Ha pensado en . . .

1 dejar el alcohol?
2 controlar el alcohol?

Have you been in . . .	Ha participado en . . .
1 detoxification?	1 desintoxicación?
2 rehabilitation?	2 rehabilitación?
3 outpatient treatment?	3 tratamiento ambulatorio?
When did you last drink alcohol?	Cuándo tomó alcohol por ultima vez?
Do you drink despite . . .	Toma alcohol aunque . . .
1 having medical problems?	1 tiene problemas médicos?
2 your doctor advising against it?	2 su médico recomienda lo contrario?
Have you ever had . . .	Ha sufrido de . . .
1 blackouts?	1 lagunas mentales?
2 hangovers?	2 resacas?
3 delirium tremens?	3 delirium tremens?
Do you use OR have you ever used . . .	Usa O ha usado . . .
1 marijuana?	1 marihuana?
2 cocaine?	2 cocaína?
3 heroin?	3 heroína?
4 LSD?	4 LSD?
5 PCP?	5 PCP?
6 mescaline?	6 mescalina?
7 amphetamines?	7 anfetamina?
8 Ecstasy?	8 Ecstasis?
9 barbiturates?	9 barbitúricos?
10 benzodiazepines?	10 benzodiacepinas?
11 cough syrup?	11 remedio para la tos?
12 sleeping pills?	12 píldoras para dormir?

15.6 ANXIETY

Do you have times when you feel nervous?

ANSIEDAD

Tiene momentos cuando se siente nervioso (a)?

When you feel nervous, do you . . .	Cuando se siente nervioso (a) sufre de . . .
1 feel shaky or tremble?	1 temblores?
2 feel tense, have sore muscles?	2 tensión o músculos dolorosos?
3 feel fidgety or can't sit still?	3 inquietud?
4 get tired easily?	4 cansancio?
5 have dry mouth?	5 la boca seca?
6 get dizzy or lightheaded?	6 mareos?
7 have cold, clammy hands?	7 las manos frías o pegajosas?
8 feel your heart beat fast?	8 palpitaciones?
9 feel like you can't catch your breath?	9 falta de aire?
10 feel you can't swallow?	10 dificultad para tragar?
11 have hot flashes/chills?	11 calores o escalofríos?
12 urinate more frequently than usual?	12 orina frecuente?
13 have trouble concentrating?	13 poca concentración?
14 jump if you hear sudden noises?	14 sustos con ruidos fuertes?
15 have trouble falling asleep?	15 dificultad para dormir?

When you feel nervous, how long do these periods last?	Cuando se siente nervioso (a), cuánto tiempo dura?
Are these periods brought on by . . .	Estos momentos ocurren cuando . . .
1 being around many people?	1 está con mucha gente?
2 being watched by others?	2 otros le miran?
3 being in certain situations . . . a heights? b around animals?	3 está en ciertas situaciones . . . a las alturas? b cerca de animales?
4 being in certain places . . .	4 está en ciertos lugares . . .
a crowded places?	a sitios que están llenos de gente?
b long lines?	b colas largas?

c buses?
d trains?
e planes?
f large parking lots?

c autobuses?
d trenes?
e aviones?
f parques de estacionamiento grandes?

Are you a nervous person?

Está nervioso (a)?

Do you worry often?

Se preocupa mucho?

Do people tell you that you worry too much?

Le dicen que se preocupa demasiado?

Are you bothered by thoughts that play in your head over and over again?

Tiene pensamientos que le ocurren repetidas veces en su mente?

Are these thoughts distressing to you?

Le molestan estos pensamientos?

Do you find it hard to control such thoughts?

Le resulta dificil controlar estos pensamientos?

Do you find you must repeat certain activities in order to reduce your distress?

Tiene que repetir ciertas actividades para bajar su angustia?

Do you find you must do things in a particular way or a particular number of times in order to feel relaxed or in order to prevent something bad from happening?

Tiene que hacer las cosas en una manera particular o cierto número de veces para sentirse cómodo (a) o para evitar que algo malo no pase?

If you can't do it the way you like or the number of times you like, do you feel . . .

Si no puede hacerlo como quisiera o el número de veces que quisiera, se siente . . .

1 anxious?
2 distressed?
3 restless?
4 irritable?

1 ansioso (a)?
2 angustiado (a)?
3 inquieto (a)?
4 irritable?

15.7 SOMATOFORM DISORDERS

Do you feel you have a serious medical condition?

Have you sought out medical evaluation?

Has it been reassuring?

When reassured that nothing is wrong, do you still worry . . .

1 about your health?
2 that the doctor missed something?

Are you bothered by many physical complaints?

Have you had a lot of trouble with . . .

1 vomiting? (when not pregnant)
2 nausea?
3 diarrhea?
4 back pain?
5 arm pain?
6 leg pain?
7 pain with urination?
8 difficulty swallowing?
9 losing your voice?
10 going blind for a short while?
11 periods of amnesia?

ENFERMEDADES SOMÁTICAS

Siente que tiene un problema médico grave?

Ha buscado evaluación médica?

Le ha dado seguridad?

Cuándo le aseguran de nuevo que todo está bien, todavía se preocupa . . .

1 por su salud?
2 que el médico le faltaba algo?

Tiene muchas molestias fisicas?

Tiene muchos problemas con . . .

1 vómitos? (cuando no está embarazada)
2 náusea?
3 diarrea?
4 dolor de espalda?
5 dolor del brazo?
6 dolor de la pierna?
7 dolor al orinar?
8 dificultad para tragar?
9 pérdida de la voz?
10 pérdida de la vista?
11 amnesia?

Appendix A
GENERAL VOCABULARY

A.1 DAYS, MONTHS, HOLIDAYS

Days of the Week[1]

Monday
Tuesday
Wednesday
Thursday
Friday
Saturday
Sunday

Dias de la Semana[1]

lunes
martes
miércoles
jueves
viernes
sábado
domingo

Months of the Year

January
February
March
April
May
June
July
August
September
October
November
December

Meses del Año

enero
febrero
marzo
abril
mayo
junio
julio
agosto
septiembre
octubre
noviembre
diciembre

[1]In Spanish, days of the week and months of the year are not capitalized.

today	hoy
yesterday	ayer
tomorrow	mañana
day before yesterday	anteayer
day after tomorrow	pasado mañana
last year	el año pasado
last month	el mes pasado
last week	la semana pasada
this year	este año
this month	este mes
this week	esta semana
next year	el año próximo
next month	el mes próximo
next week	la semana próxima

Holidays   **Días de Fiesta**

Christmas	Navidad
New Year	Año Nuevo
Valentine's Day	Día de San Valentín
Easter	Pascua
Holy Week	Semana Santa
July 4	Cuatro de julio
Halloween	Día de todos los Santos
birthday	cumpleaños
anniversary	aniversario

A.2 CARDINAL AND ORDINAL NUMBERS

NÚMEROS CARDINALES Y ORDINALES

Cardinal Numbers

1	uno	9	nueve
2	dos	10	diez
3	tres	11	once
4	cuatro	12	doce
5	cinco	13	trece
6	seis	14	catorce
7	siete	15	quince
8	ocho	20	veinte

30	treinta	80	ochenta
40	cuarenta	90	noventa
50	cincuenta	100	cien
60	sesenta	1000	mil
70	setenta	1,000,000	millón

Other numbers are made by adding two numbers

10 + 6	diez y seis or dieciseis
10 + 7	diez y siete or diecisiete
20 + 1	veinte y uno or veintiuno

Ordinal Numbers

first	primero (a)	seventh	séptimo (a)
second	segundo (a)	eighth	octavo (a)
third	tercero (a)	ninth	noveno (a)
fourth	cuarto (a)	tenth	décimo (a)
fifth	quinto (a)	eleventh	undécimo
sixth	sexto (a)	twelfth	duodécimo

A.3 TIME EXPRESSIONS

EXPRESIONES DEL TIEMPO

hour	hora
minute	minuto
second	segundo
at noon	al mediodía
at midnight	a la medianoche
in the morning[2,3]	por la mañana,[2] durante la mañana[3]
in the afternoon	por la tarde, durante la tarde
in the evening	por la noche, durante la noche

The word "time" has three translations

1   What TIME is it?   Qué HORA es?

[2]When "in" is translated as "por," the expression refers to "morning" as a short interval of time, no specific hour.
[3]When "in" is translated as "durante," the expression refers to "morning" as a larger interval of time, but still no specific hour.

In this instance "time" is translated as "hora" (hour).

2 Take the medicine three   Tome la medicina tres
   TIMES a day.   VECES al día.

Here the word "time" refers to time in a series. It is used for a repeated action. ("Vez" is the singular form of "veces.")

3 I have TIME to see you   Tengo TIEMPO para verle
   today.   hoy.

"Tiempo" is used to express time in the sense of duration.

What time is it?   Qué hora es?

Between the hour and the half hour, *add* the number of minutes to the hour.

Example:

It is 3:00 in the afternoon.[4]   Son las tres de la *tarde*.[4]
It is 3:10. (It is 3 AND 10.)   Son las tres Y diez.
It is 3:30.[5]   Son las tres *y media*.[5]
It is 3:15.[6]   Son las tres *y cuarto*.[6]

Between the half hour and the next hour, *subtract* the number of minutes from the next hour.

Example:

It is 3:40: (it is 4 MINUS 20.)   Son las cuatro MENOS veinte.

It is 3:45.   Son las cuatro menos cuarto.

It is 3:55.   Son las cuatro menos cinco.

The third-person plural form of the verb "ser" (to be) is "son." When telling time, this form is used with every hour except 1 o'clock, for which the singular form "es" is used.

Example:

It is 1:00.   Es la una.

---

[4]When a specific hour is given,
in the morning
in the afternoon   are translated as
in the evening
de la mañana
de la tarde
de la noche
[5]*media*: one-half, 30 minutes.
[6]*cuarto*: one-quarter, 15 minutes.

It is 1:20.
It is 1:30.
It is 12:50.

Es la una y veinte.
Es la una y media.
Es la una menos diez.

A.4 COLORS

What color is it?
red
white
green
blue
black
brown
gray
yellow
purple
pink

COLORES

De qué color es?
rojo (a)
blanco (a)
verde
azul
negro (a)
café
gris
amarillo (a)
morado (a)
rosado (a)

A.5 CONTRASTING ADJECTIVES

large
small

tall (for height)
short (for height)

high
low

long (for length)
short (for length)

fat
thin

heavy (for weight)
light (for weight)

dark (for colors)
light (for colors)

ADJETIVOS QUE CONTRASTAN

grande
pequeño (a)

alto (a)
bajo (a)

alto (a)
bajo (a)

largo (a)
corto (a)

gordo (a)
flaco (a), delgado (a),
seco (a)

pesado (a)
liviano (a), ligero (a)

oscuro (a)
claro (a)

round	redondo (a)
square	cuadrado (a)
rectangular	rectangular
triangular	triangular
oval	ovalado (a)
smooth	liso (a)
rough	áspero (a), rugoso (a)
regular	regular
irregular	irregular
curly	rizado (a), crespo (a)
straight	liso (a)
soft	suave
hard	duro (a)
tepid	tibio (a)
hot	caliente
boiling	hirviendo
wet	mojado
dry	seco (a)
humid	húmedo (a)
open	abierto (a)
closed	cerrado (a)
painful	doloroso (a)
painless	sin dolor
many	muchos (as)
some	algunos (as)
few	pocos (as)
mobile	móvil
immobile	inmóvil
flat	plano (a)
raised	elevado (a)
central	central
peripheral	periférico (a)

loud	fuerte
soft	suave
weak	débil
strong	fuerte
symmetric	simétrico (a)
asymmetric	asimétrico (a)
better	mejor
worse	peor
the best	lo mejor
the worst	lo peor
alive	vivo (a)
dead	muerto (a)
healthy	sano (a) ,
sick	enfermo (a)
sweet	dulce
sour	agrio (a)
bitter	amargo (a)

A.6 WEIGHTS AND MEASURES

PESOS Y MEDIDAS

length	longitud
width	ancho
height	altura
volume	volumen
weight	peso
gram	gramo
kilogram	kilogramo
liter	litro
square millimeter	milímetro cuadrado .
square centimeter	centímetro cuadrado
cubic centimeter	centímetro cúbico
millimeter	milímetro
centimeter	centímetro
milligram	miligramo
microgram	microgramo

A.7 PHRASES FOR THE FIRST VISIT

Come in please.
My name is ____.
I am the doctor.
I am the nurse.
I am the assistant.
Who is the patient?
What is your name?
It's nice to meet you.
Did you come alone?
Who brought you?
I would like to talk to you now.
Later I will examine you.

EXPRESIONES PARA LA PRIMERA VISITA

Entre, por favor.
Me llamo ____.
Soy doctor.
Soy enfermera (o).
Soy asistente.
Quién es el paciente?
Cómo se llama?
Mucho gusto en conocerle.
Vino solo (a)?
Quién le trajo?
Me gustaría hablar con usted ahora.
Más tarde le voy a examinar.

Appendix B
COMMONLY
REQUESTED
TESTS

amniocentesis	amniocentesis
anesthesia	anestesia
angiogram	angiograma
angioplasty	angioplastía
arthrogram	arthrograma
arthroscopy	artroscopía
audiogram	audiograma
barium enema	enema de bario
biopsy	biopsia
blood gas	gasometría
blood test	prueba de sangre
bone-marrow biopsy	biopsia de la médula ósea
bronchoscopy	broncoscopía
CAT scan	tomografía computada
catheterization, cardiac	cateterismo cardíaco
checkup	chequeo
cholangiogram . . .	colangiograma . . .
endoscopic	endoscópico
percutaneous	percutáneo
colonoscopy	colonoscopía
colposcopy	colposcopía
cystoscopy	cistoscopía
dilatation and curettage	dilatación y legrado
drainage	drenaje

electrocardiogram	electrocardiograma
electroencephalogram	electroencefalograma
electromyography	electromiografía
endoscopic retrograde	colangiopancreatografía
cholangiopancreatography	retrógrada endoscópica
(ERCP)	
endoscopic ultrasound	ultrasonido endoscópico
endoscopy	endoscopía
fluoroscopy	fluroscopía
intravenous pyelogram	pielograma intravenoso
laparoscopy	laparoscopía
laryngoscopy	laringoscopía
magnetic resonance imaging	imágenes por resonancia
scan (MRI)	magnética
mammogram	mamografía
manometry	manometría
monitor . . .	monitor . . .
cardiac	cardíaco
fetal	cardíaco fetal
holter	cardíaco ambulatorio
myelogram	mielograma
Pap smear	examen de Papanicolaou
retrograde pyelogram	pielograma retrógrado
sigmoidoscopy (flexible)	sigmoidoscopía (flexible)
slit-lamp	lámpara de hendidura
sonogram	sonograma
spirometry	espirometría
tomography . . .	tomografía . . .
CT	computada
PET	por emisión de positrones
ultrasound	ultrasonido
urinalysis	examen de orina
urography . . .	urografía . . .
excretory	excretoria
retrograde	retrograda
venogram	venograma
x-ray	radiografía

Appendix C
COUNTRIES OF
THE WORLD

COUNTRIES OF THE WORLD	PAISES DEL MUNDO
Afghanistan	Afganistán
Albania	Albania
Angola	Angola
Anguilla	Anguilla
Argentina	Argentina
Aruba	Aruba
Australia	Australia
Austria	Austria
Bahamas	Bahamas
Bahrain	Bahrein
Bangladesh	Bangladesh
Barbados	Barbados
Belgium	Bélgica
Belize	Belice
Bermuda	Bermuda
Bhutan	Bhutan
Bolivia	Bolivia
Botswana	Botswana
Brazil	Brasil
British Virgin Island	Islas Virgenes Británicas
Bulgaria	Bulgaria
Cambodia	Camboya
Cameron	Camerún
Canada	Canadá

Cayman Islands	Islas Caimanes
Chile	Chile
China	China
Colombia	Colombia
Costa Rica	Costa Rica
Croatia	Croacia
Cuba	Cuba
Cyprus	Chipre
Czech Republic	República Checa
Denmark	Dinamarca
Dominica	Dominica
Dominican Republic	República Dominicana
Ecuador	Ecuador
Egypt	Egipto
El Salvador	El Salvador
Equatorial Guinea	Guinea Ecuatorial
Ethiopia	Etiopía
Fiji	Fiji
Finland	Finlandia
France	Francia
French Guyana	Guayana Francesa
French Polynesia	Polinesia Francesa
Gambia	Gambia
Germany	Alemania
Ghana	Ghana
Gibraltar	Gibraltar
Greece	Grecia
Guatemala	Guatemala
Haiti	Haití
Holland	Holanda
Honduras	Honduras
Hong Kong	Hong Kong
Hungary	Hungría
Iceland	Irlanda
India	India
Indonesia	Indonesia
Iran	Irán
Iraq	Irak
Ireland	Irlanda

Israel	Israel
Italy	Italia
Jamaica	Jamaica
Japan	Japón
Jordan	Jordania
Kenya	Kenia
Laos	Laos
Liberia	Liberia
Libya	Libia
Lithuania	Lituania
Luxembourg	Luxemburgo
Malaysia	Malasia
Marshall Island	Marshall Islas
Martinique	Martinica
Mexico	México
Monaco	Mónaco
Mongolia	Mongolia
Morocco	Marruecos
Mozambique	Mozambique
Namibia	Namibia
Nepal	Nepal
New Zealand	Nueva Zelandia
Nicaragua	Nicaragua
Nigeria	Nigeria
North Korea	Corea del Norte
Norway	Noruega
Pakistan	Pakistán
Panama	Panamá
Paraguay	Paraguay
Peru	Perú
Philippines	Filipinas
Poland	Polonia
Portugal	Portugal
Puerto Rico	Puerto Rico
Qatar	Qatar
Rumania	Rumania
Russia	Rusia
Saudi Arabia	Arabia Saudita
Senegal	Senegal

Sierra Leone	Sierra Leona
Singapore	Singapur
Somalia	Somalia
South Africa	Sudáfrica
South Korea	Corea del Sur
Spain	España
Sri Lanka	Sri Lanka
Sudan	Sudán
Swaziland	Swazilandia
Sweden	Suecia
Switzerland	Suiza
Syria	Siria
Taiwan	Taiwán
Tanzania	Tanzania
Thailand	Tailandia
Tunis	Túnez
Turkey	Turquía
Uganda	Uganda
Ukraine	Ucrania
United Arab Emirates	Emiratos Arabes Unidos
United States of America	Estados Unidos de América
Uruguay	Uruguay
US Virgin Islands	Islas Virgenes Americanas
Vatican City	Ciudad del Vaticano
Venezuela	Venezuela
Vietnam	Vietnam
Yemen	Yemen
Zambia	Zambia
Zimbabwe	Zimbabwe

INDEX OF TERMS

Some terms in this index appear without page numbers. They are included, with the Spanish translation, for reference purposes. An index of verbs follows this index.

191

INDEX OF VERBS